II

Repressed Memories

I

pressed
emories

Section II

Repressed Memories

Foreword

David Spiegel, M.D., Section Editor

Can those subjected to traumatic stressors forget to remember? Is traumatic memory too malleable to be trusted or too accurate to be avoided? The discussion and exploration of memory in psychotherapy has become a traumatic topic in itself in recent years. Prominent court cases involving recovered memories of sexual abuse and even murder have brought the phenomenon to national attention. Some doubt the veracity of any repressed memory, and others insist that the very absence of memory proves that a traumatic event occurred. These issues are at the heart of psychotherapy, the daily currency of which is the mining and working through of memories, be they of childhood experience, trauma, recent stressors, relationship problems, or existential dread. Memory is a complex but remarkable aspect of mental function, allowing us to organize a huge amount of information. Affect helps us do this, labeling certain memories as critically important and others as forgettable. However, the evidence reviewed below suggests that emotion may have other effects on memory and that the very association between mood and memory may make the regulation of conscious retrieval of memories a means of managing uncomfortable emotion. The authors examine both the research and clinical literature, providing evidence that memory of trauma is less than perfect but more than fantasy. Those who have experienced trauma and those who treat these people must come to grips with the vagaries and accuracies of memory.

In Chapter 6 (Butler and Spiegel), we examine the relationship between laboratory research on memory in cognitive psychology and clinical investigation of traumatic amnesia and other memory impairments. Mr. Justice Frankfurter once warned against the "cross-sterilization of disciplines." We caution that certain questionable assumptions underlie the facile application of laboratory findings to clinical problems: 1) the continuum fallacy: that childhood sexual abuse is simply more stressful than watching an upsetting movie; 2) the population generalizability problem: that college undergraduates provide findings salient to clinical populations; and 3) the difference between what is reported and what is remembered. Furthermore, we argue that a false dichotomy has been constructed in the literature using laboratory studies of suggested misinformation to argue that memory is unreliable and therefore, in particular, that repressed memories are suggested memories. After reviewing literature documenting repression of traumatic memories, we point out that suggested intrusion of false memory is the other side of the coin of suggested repression of real memory. Indeed, recent misinformation research has provided laboratory models of repression of real, if minor, traumatic memory. We argue that the nature of traumatic dissociative amnesia is such that it is not subject to the same rules of ordinary forgetting: it is more, rather than less, common after repeated episodes; involves strong affect; and is resistant to retrieval through salient cues. Laboratory research shows that stressful affect generally enhances memory for central information at the expense of peripheral details. In contrast to this general rule, dissociative amnesia involves central and peripheral information. We find that laboratory investigators are moving in the direction of assessing clinical problems, and clinicians are seeking systematic information with independent verification of memories. Both are salutary directions and should move the field toward the resolution of apparent contradictions.

In Chapter 7, Dr. McConkey points out that the laboratory and the clinic are complementary rather than competing venues. He notes that repressed memories can be distorted in the same way that non-repressed memories can. The fact that repressed memories are not completely accurate does not render them completely inaccurate. He notes that trauma affects cognitive function when it occurs and may affect brain systems afterward, as research showing reduced size of the hippocampus in veterans with posttraumatic stress disorder indicates. Thus, distortion of one cognitive function—memory—in the aftermath of trauma is not surprising. He reviews literature documenting memory distortion or amnesia for traumatic events. His own work has demonstrated that suggestive effects of memory retrieval facilitators such as hypnosis may affect confidence in memory more than content, producing "confident errors." He recommends that therapists be cautious about either accepting or rejecting memories of trauma and that more research be devoted to the usefulness of memory retrieval in the psychotherapy of posttraumatic stress syndromes.

In Chapter 8, by Koutstaal and Schacter, we are treated to a thorough and thoughtful examination of an aspect of memory processing and trauma that is often overlooked. The debate often involves two relatively discontinuous analyses of the response to trauma: such memories either are not likely to be forgotten, or, if they are not remembered, they did not happen. In this chapter, the authors explore the middle ground. It is not at all uncommon, as the authors note, for people to use various strategies to avoid thinking about trauma. They make dramatic moves—staying with a friend, changing apartments, or even leaving town—as a way of removing themselves from clues that will trigger memories of a rape. Koutstaal and Schacter remind us that such strategies work with varying degrees of success. Under certain circumstances, people can reduce the frequency with which they recall information by simply instructing themselves to forget. However, in some circumstances, particularly with neutral information, there tends to be a rebound—a return of the suppressed—and they remember it more later on. This may come from cue contamination, when people distract themselves from the memory to be avoided but wind up creating associations to the distracters. The authors note that a particularly unsuccessful strategy is often used by depressed individuals, who find themselves avoiding one depressive contact by focusing on another one, which produces an affective link that may stimulate cued recall. However, the experimental literature suggests that neutral stimuli are more likely to rebound than emotional stimuli. Of course, the kind of emotional triggers that one can mobilize in the laboratory are far different in intensity and even valence from those that one sees clinically in the aftermath of trauma.

The instincts of a psychotherapist are quite consistent with their observation at the end of Chapter 8 that the most effective suppression of thought may well come with its initial expression. This finding provides experimental support for the idea of critical incident debriefing after trauma and for more traditional psychotherapy. This chapter is an important contribution to the developing literature on effects of traumatic stress on memory and provides a useful bridge between conscious strategies enacted to control traumatic memories and the traditional literature on defense mechanisms.

In Chapter 9, Williams and Banyard review research on traumatic amnesia, noting the logical necessity that patients have both true and false memories of the presence and absence of abuse. That is, if it is possible to construct a false memory that abuse happened when it did not, it also must be possible to construct a false memory that abuse did not happen when in fact it did. Williams's own important research provided evidence that a substantial minority of women with documented histories of abuse requiring an emergency room visit did not recall the episode some 17 years later. They have thus shown that amnesia for real episodes occurs. This amnesia is not always continuous, and many women did recall the episode (although not necessarily continuously from the time it happened). In their chapter, the theme of the previous one is amplified, noting that forgetting of trauma may well be more than the aftermath of a conscious strategy of suppression, although it may derive from that as well.

In Chapter 10, Coons and colleagues provide a useful and important review of the clinical literature on traumatic amnesia. They point out that memory gaps are not uncommon in the aftermath of traumatic stressors, ranging from incest to the Holocaust. They provide data showing that histories of sexual and physical abuse in childhood are far more common among patients with dissociative disorders than in those with affective disorders. Traumatic amnesia occurred in both groups but was far more common among patients with dissociative disorder. The authors make a series of sensible and practical recommendations regarding memory in the psychotherapy of patients with recovered memories of trauma. These recommendations are very much in keeping with the American Psychiatric Association's Statement on Memories of Sexual Abuse, referred to in Chapter 7. This statement is well thought out, sensible, and practical. Much support for it can be found in the chapters in this section, and, for this reason, I include it below:

Statement on Memories of Sexual Abuse[1]

This *Statement* is in response to the growing concern regarding memories of sexual abuse. The rise in reports of documented cases of child sexual abuse has been accompanied by a rise in reports of sexual abuse that cannot be documented. Members of the public, as well as members of mental health and other professions, have debated the validity of some memories of sexual abuse, as well as some of the therapeutic techniques which have been used. The American Psychiatric Association has been concerned that the passionate debates about these issues have obscured the recognition of a body of scientific evidence that underlies widespread agreement among psychiatrists regarding psychiatric treatment in this area. We are especially concerned that the public confusion and dismay over this issue and the possibility of false accusations not discredit the reports of patients who have indeed been traumatized by actual previous abuse. While much more needs to be known, this *Statement* summarizes information about this topic that is important for psychiatrists in their work with patients for whom sexual abuse is an issue.

Sexual abuse of children and adolescents leads to severe negative consequences. Child sexual abuse is a risk factor for many classes of psychiatric disorders, including anxiety disorders, affective disorders, dissociative disorders and personality disorders.

Children and adolescents may be abused by family members, including parents and siblings, and by individuals outside of their families, including adults in trusted positions (e.g., teachers, clergy, camp counsellors). Abusers come from all walks of life. There is no uniform "profile" or other method to accurately distinguish those who have sexually abused children from those who have not.

Children and adolescents who have been abused cope with trauma by using a variety of psychological mechanisms. In some instances, these coping mechanisms result in a lack of conscious awareness of the abuse for varying periods of time. Conscious thoughts and feelings stemming from the abuse may emerge at a later date.

It is not known how to distinguish, with complete accuracy, memories based on true events from those derived from other sources. The following observations have been made:

- Human memory is a complex process about which there is a substantial base of scientific knowledge. Memory can be divided into four stages: input (encoding), storage, retrieval, and recounting. All of these processes can be influenced by a variety of factors, including developmental stage, expectations and knowledge base prior to an event; stress and bodily sensations experienced during an event; post-event questioning; and the experience and context of the recounting of the event. In addition, the retrieval and recounting of a memory can modify the form of the memory, which may influence the content and the conviction about the veracity of the memory in the future. Scientific knowledge is not yet precise enough to predict how a certain experience or factor will influence a memory in a given person.
- Implicit and explicit memory are two different forms of memory that have been identified. *Explicit memory* (also termed declarative memory) refers to the ability to consciously recall facts or events. *Implicit memory* (also termed procedural memory) refers to behavioral knowledge of an experience without conscious recall. A child who demonstrates knowledge of a skill (e.g., bicycle riding) without recalling how he/she learned it, or an adult who has an affective reaction (e.g., a combat veteran who panics when he hears the sound of a helicopter, but cannot remember that he was in a helicopter crash which killed his best friend) are demonstrating implicit memories in the absence of explicit recall. This distinction between explicit and implicit memory is fundamental because they have been shown to be supported by different brain systems, and because their differentiation and identification may have important clinical implications.
- Some individuals who have experienced documented traumatic events may nevertheless include some false or inconsistent elements in their reports. In addition, hesitancy in making a report, and recanting following the report can occur in victims of documented abuse. Therefore, these seemingly contradictory findings do not exclude the possibility that the report is based on a true event.
- Memories can be significantly influenced by questioning, especially in young children. Memories also can be significantly influenced by

a trusted person (e.g., therapist, parent involved in a custody dispute) who suggests symptoms/problems, despite initial lack of memory of such abuse. It has also been shown that repeated questioning may lead individuals to report "memories" of events that never occurred.

It is not known what proportion of adults who report memories of sexual abuse were actually abused. Many individuals who recover memories of sexual abuse have been able to find corroborating information about their memories. However, no such information can be found, or is possible to obtain, in some situations. While aspects of the alleged abuse situation, as well as the context in which the memories emerge, can contribute to the assessment, there is no completely accurate way of determining the validity of reports in the absence of corroborating information.

Psychiatrists are often consulted in situation in which memories of sexual abuse are critical issues. Psychiatrists may be involved in a variety of capacities, including as the treating clinician for the alleged victim, for the alleged abuser, or for other family member(s); as a school consultant; or in a forensic capacity.

Basic clinical and ethical principles should guide the psychiatrist's work in this difficult area. These include the need for role clarity. It is essential that the psychiatrist and the other involved parties understand and agree on the psychiatrist's role.

Psychiatrists should maintain an empathic, nonjudgmental, neutral stance towards reported memories of sexual abuse. As in the treatment of all patients, care must be taken to avoid prejudging the cause of the patient's difficulties, or the veracity of the patient's reports. A strong prior belief by the psychiatrist that sexual abuse, or other factors, are or are not the cause of the patient's problems is likely to interfere with appropriate assessment and treatment. Many individuals who have experienced sexual abuse have a history of not being believed by their parents, or other in whom they have put their trust. Expression of disbelief is likely to cause the patient further pain and decrease his/her willingness to seek needed psychiatric treatment. Similarly, clinicians should not exert pressure on patients to believe in events that may not have occurred, or to prematurely disrupt important relationships or make other important decisions based on these speculations. Clinicians who have not had the training necessary to evaluate and treat patients with a broad range of psychiatric disorders are at risk of causing harm by providing inadequate care for the patient's problems and by increasing the patient's resistance to obtaining and responding to appropriate treatment in the future. In addition, special knowledge and experience are necessary to properly evaluate and/or treat patients who report the emergence of memories during the use of specialized techniques (e.g., the use of hypnosis or amytal), or during the course of litigation.

The treatment plan should be based on a complete psychiatric assessment, and should address the full range of the patient's clinical needs. In addition to specific treatments for any primary psychiatric condition, the patient may need help recognizing and integrating data that informs and defines the issue related to the memories of abuse. As in the treatment of patients with any psychiatric disorder, it may be important to caution the patient against making major life decisions during the acute phase of treatment. During the acute and later phases of treatment, the issues of breaking off relationships with important attachment figures, of pursuing legal actions, and of making public disclosures may need to be addressed. The psychiatrist should help the patient assess the likely impact (including emotional) of such decisions, given the patient's overall clinical and social situation. Some patients will be left with unclear memories of abuse and no corroborating information. Psychiatric treatment may help these patients adapt to the uncertainty regarding such emotionally important issues.

The intensity of public interest and debate about these topics should not influence psychiatrists to abandon their commitment to basic principles of ethical practice, delineated in *The Principles of Medical Ethics With Annotations Especially Applicable to Psychiatry*. The following concerns are of particular relevance:

- Psychiatrists should refrain from making public statements about the veracity or other features of individual reports of sexual abuse.
- Psychiatrists should vigilantly assess the impact of the conduct on the boundaries of the doctor/patient relationship. This is especially critical when treating patients who are seeking care for conditions that are associated with boundary violations in their past.

The APA will continue to monitor developments in this area in an effort to help psychiatrists provide the best possible care for their patients.

This statement was approved by the Board of Trustees of the American Psychiatric Association on December 12, 1993.

Chapter 6

Trauma and Memory

Lisa D. Butler, Ph.D., and David Spiegel, M.D.

We forget because we must
And not because we will.

Matthew Arnold, "Switzerland,"
Empedocles on Etna, and Other Poems (1852)

The debate over memories of traumatic experience has itself become a traumatic experience for clinicians, patients, family members, and researchers. Increasingly, it has come to pit therapists, trauma survivors, and researchers on child abuse against families, sociologists, and researchers on memory. As is often the case in such situations, each side has come to take a rather one-dimensional view of the other. The "recovered memory" movement sees criticism as a shield behind which child abusers hide, whereas the "false memory" movement accuses psychotherapists of using their professional credentials as a hunting license, with family reputations being fair game.

This issue is too important to be left to the domain of accusation. The very concept of psychotherapy is built on the reexamination of memories. Classic psychoanalytic and modern psychodynamic psychotherapy—not just so-called recovered memory therapy—assume that current problems may reflect memories of life experiences, such as traumatic events (incest, assault, accidents), family stresses, or warded-off fears and wishes, which may be only partially accessible to consciousness at a given time. In some cases, people simply may not connect an available memory with a symptom; in other cases, they may not consciously remember the event. Consequently, many of the essential elements of psychotherapy—transference, working through, and re-

The authors wish to thank Elizabeth Bowman, M.D., Robert Garlan, A.B., and Cheryl Koopman, Ph.D., for their extremely helpful suggestions on earlier versions of this manuscript. The authors also express their great appreciation to Gordon Bower, Ph.D., for his critical reading of the manuscript and his extensive and invaluable recommendations for its improvement.

Supported by a National Institute of Mental Health National Research Service Award MH-19908 (L. D. B.) and a grant from the John D. and Catherine T. MacArthur Foundation (D. S.).

structuring—involve working with memories. The need for psychotherapy, in turn, is greater when individuals have had traumatic experiences. Psychotherapy remains the primary treatment for trauma victims, with pharmacological agents playing only a secondary role (Krystal et al., in press; Maldonado and Spiegel 1994). Understanding the effects of trauma on memory is critical to the therapeutic use of memory to affect the aftermath of trauma. Thus, this issue is of great practical and theoretical importance.

Fortunately, both experimental and clinical research offer considerable bodies of knowledge to inform our understanding of the effects of trauma on memory. However, they represent two distinct research traditions, and much of the debate that has arisen between them may be seen, at least in part, as a function of their differing perspectives. Experimental cognitive psychology and clinical psychology and psychiatry differ in so many fundamental respects that they often seem to inhabit different countries and speak different languages. Indeed, they actually study different populations, operate at different levels of analysis, use different tools, and proceed from quite different assumptions. These differences and their consequences must be considered in any analysis of the applicability of the findings of experimental research to clinical phenomena.

In this chapter, we focus on two broad areas: the effects of traumatic experience on memory and the status of laboratory findings of memory alteration and implantation as a model to explain recovered memories. We begin by briefly discussing problems in generalizing experimental research to clinical issues. As an example, we note that although cognitive research with nonclinical subjects has found that negative emotion tends to enhance memory for central details, there is evidence of significant memory disturbance in populations of trauma survivors. We also examine several of the explanations for traumatic amnesia offered by cognitive psychologists, emphasizing critical features that are not accounted for. Next, we describe the cognitive laboratory demonstrations of memory alteration and implantation in nonclinical subjects (known as misinformation effects) and outline some of the limitations of these effects relative to claims made about them. Then, we briefly discuss what the recent memory implantation findings may tell us about recovered memories. We propose that these findings are not inconsistent with a mechanism of dissociation to explain traumatic amnesia and recovered memories, and we argue that they may even be viewed as evidence in support of it. The following is necessarily a selective examination of these topics—we highlight issues that we believe are particularly important, especially to the currently polarized debate about repressed memories.

A few words about terminology are in order. We use the term *traumatic event* to refer to events that would be expected to evoke feelings of fear, helplessness, or horror and involve actual or threatened injury or threat to the physical integrity of self or others (see American Psychiatric Association 1994, pp. 427–428). Our use of the term *traumatic amnesia* implies many of the characteristics of the diagnostic term *dissociative amnesia* (American Psychiatric Association 1994). That is, it refers to a potentially reversible memory impairment characterized by an inability to recall important personal information of a traumatic or stressful nature and that seems too extensive to be explained by normal forgetfulness. Because diagnostic criteria have not been formally applied in most reported cases, we have chosen to use the general descriptive term rather than the specific diagnostic one. Use of the term *traumatic memories* is somewhat more complicated. In general, we use it to refer to memories of traumatic events. However, in some of the clinical literature, the term denotes specific types of posttraumatic memory disturbances such as intrusive memories (e.g., van der Kolk and van der Hart 1991). We have tried to point out when this change in usage occurs. Unfortunately, often there is little general agreement on terminology within disciplines and even less between them. Consequently, much of the clinical and experimental research described in this chapter employs different terms or similar terms with different meanings. Rather than trying to impose our definitions on these reports, we have elected in many cases to retain original terms.

Traumatic Memory and Amnesia

Before proceeding to a specific discussion of the effects of negative emotion on memory, we briefly review a number of the properties of memory that are relevant to an understanding of the effects of trauma on memory (for a more comprehensive review, see L. D. Butler, R. W. Garlan, D. Spiegel, "Some things experimental cognitive psychology can and cannot tell us about trauma and memory," unpublished manuscript, November 1996; Siegel 1995). First, the distinction between explicit and implicit memory (Schacter 1992; Squire 1992) suggests that experiences of abuse may be recorded—and then recalled and expressed—by different means (i.e., conscious/narrative vs. nonconscious/behavioral; Siegel 1995). Moreover, explicit adult autobiographical memory tends not to extend to events experienced during preverbal childhood (Nelson 1993), so caution should be used in considering narrative reports of memory from that period. Behavioral (implicit) memories, on the other hand, do not appear to be subject to infantile amnesia (Schacter and Moscovitch 1984) and therefore may be more reliable indicators of early childhood abuse (Terr 1988).

In addition, the processing of experience into memory is affected by a number of factors, including the degree to which it is elaborated, organized, and rehearsed (Kihlstrom 1994). In the case of sexual abuse, cognitive avoidance strategies (Bower 1990; see also Koutstaal and Schacter, Chapter 8, in this volume) or environmental prohibitions against verbalizing and sharing such information (Freyd 1993) may therefore undermine encoding, storage, and/or retrieval of these memories. Explicit memory, whether it be of generic event schemata or specific autobiographical episodes, may also be unwittingly influenced by vicariously learned information (e.g., Pynoos and Nader 1989). Consequently, one may have relatively elaborate cognitive structures for events that have not been personally experienced. Recovery of memories of childhood abuse is often precipitated by some environmental cue or trigger (Elliot and Fox 1994; Feldman-Summers and Pope 1994), and, in general, this appears consistent with the central role of cues in normal recall (Bower 1990; Kihlstrom 1994). Normal memory is undeniably reconstructive and imperfect (Bartlett 1932), with the clinical implication that findings of errors or inconsistencies in the recall of abuse experiences need not cast doubt on the central truth of the memory, any more than would be the case for nonabuse memories. However, confidence in a memory should not be taken as a reliable reflection of the truth of the memory (for a discussion, see Lindsay and Read 1994). With this background, we can begin our discussion of the cognitive literature on affect and recall.

Effects of Negative Affect on Recall: Cognitive Psychological Data

The literature describing the effects of emotion on memory is extensive, encompassing a number of research approaches that examine personal memories of negative or traumatic events, personal memories of significant public events ("flashbulb memories"), and memories of simulated negative events (shown on slides, videotapes, or staged) in laboratory settings. In the recent literature on memories of negative events, the general consensus is that such events seem to be better remembered than neutral events, and within negative events, central details or themes are better remembered than peripheral and contextual information (for an extensive review of memory for negative emotional events, see Christianson 1992).

Emotion and recall of details.   In studies of the characteristics of naturally occurring memories of negative emotional ("traumatic") events in college populations (Christianson and Loftus 1990; Wessel and Merckelbach 1994), subjects report remembering more central than peripheral details, and the degree of emotion at the time of the event tends to be positively correlated with the amount of central, but not always peripheral, detail information that is remembered.

These findings are similar to the "weapon focus" effect (Loftus et al. 1987) reported by victims of and witnesses to crimes. Their descriptions suggest that one's attention during a crime is so focused on the weapon that little else is attended to; thus, poor recall of other details of the environment or event may be expected. The highly stressful nature of the situation presumably results in a narrowing of the range of the perceptual field, enhancing memory for the limited information attended to at the expense of information outside the range of this focus (Burke et al. 1992; Easterbrook 1959; for a discussion, see Christianson 1992). In the clinical literature, this phenomenon is also described in altered states of consciousness, such as during formal hypnosis or dissociative states (see Butler et al. 1996; D. Spiegel and Cardeña 1990). Termed *absorption*, it represents a state of highly focused attention (D. Spiegel 1992; Tellegen 1981; Tellegen and Atkinson 1974), which results in the exclusion of other experience or perceptual data that normally may be present in conscious awareness. This constriction of focus relegates other perceptual inputs to the periphery of consciousness, where they receive considerably less, if any, conscious cognitive processing and, therefore, are not committed to memory or may be more difficult to retrieve.

Emotion and accuracy.   In addition to determining the primacy of recall for central versus peripheral details, when the facts about an event are known, memories may also be assessed for accuracy. In a study of actual witnesses to robberies, Christianson and Hubinette (1993) found relatively accurate memories for details associated with the robbery itself (action, weapon, clothing of the robber) but lower accuracy for other details (such as time, date, eye color of robber). In addition, higher accuracy rates were found for victims when compared with bystanders, although, surprisingly, different levels of emotion were not associated with differences in recollection.

The accuracy of personal memories for potentially upsetting public events has also been studied. *Flashbulb memory* (R. Brown and Kulik 1977; Pillemer 1984) is a term used to describe a vivid memory of a significant newsworthy event (e.g., learning of the Challenger explosion or the assassination of John F. Kennedy) and the circumstances surrounding learning of it (such as who told you, where you were, what you were doing, what time of day it was). Although the implication of the label is that a near-perfect "photographic" memory for the experience is retained, this has not been supported by all investigations (McCloskey et al. 1988; Neisser 1982). Nonetheless, Christianson (1992, p. 288) observed that "the loss of clarity and detail over time seems to be far less for these emotional memories than can be seen from the forgetting curve typically found in basic memory research (Murdock 1974)."

Laboratory studies of memory for emotional events have also produced mixed findings; however, Christianson (1992) concluded in his review of this literature that these findings are consistent overall with findings regarding memory for emotional events in real life. In one series of laboratory studies, Christianson and Loftus (1987) asked subjects to view slides/video of a traumatic event (e.g., witnessing someone being hit by a car or being shot during a bank robbery) or a neutral version of the same event. In the slide studies, subjects were instructed to pay close attention and rehearse the central detail of each slide (they wrote down a descriptive word). Subjects' memories were then tested after short (20 minutes) or longer (2 weeks) retention intervals. The results suggested that subjects who viewed the traumatic event were better able to remember the central details than those who viewed the neutral event. However, the traumatic group was less able to recognize the specific slides they had seen (they were varied by camera angle), indicating that memory was impaired in this group for some of the specific details, especially peripheral details (see also Burke et al. 1992). When tested again at 6 months, subjects who had initially viewed the traumatic event were more likely to recall the essence or theme of the event than subjects who had initially viewed the neutral event (see also Burke et al. 1992).

Because laboratory studies are controlled, they offer opportunities to study additional factors. For example, such studies have found that shocking events may impair memory for details present before the emotion-arousing event (Loftus and Burns 1982). In addition, some high-arousal events may be equally or less well remembered than low-arousal events at short retention intervals (which adds to some of the mixed findings in laboratory studies), but memory performance tends to be superior for high-arousal events compared with low-arousal events when testing intervals are delayed (Christianson 1992).

In summary, the cognitive literature on negative mood and memory, which includes studies of personal memories of negative or traumatic events, personal memories of significant public events (flashbulb memories), and memories of simulated negative events in laboratory settings, suggests that "highly negative events are relatively well retained, both with respect to the emotional event itself and with respect to the central critical information of the emotion-eliciting event—the information that elicits the emotional reaction" (Christianson 1992, p. 303). It is appropriate, then, to consider the degree to which these findings apply to clinical phenomena.

Application of Laboratory Research to the Clinical World

Bannister (1966, p. 24) noted that "in order to behave like scientists we must construct situations in which our subjects . . . can behave as little like human beings as possible and we do this in order to allow ourselves to make statements about the nature of their humanity." Just as dissection requires sacrifice of the living nature of the creature in favor of isolating and describing its physical components, so the controlled experimental study of human behavior often requires that it be plucked from its natural context and stripped of its rich, dynamic character to reveal basic processes and mechanisms.

This observation may have implications for the conclusions we may reasonably draw from experimental research. Campbell and Stanley introduced the concept of external validity three decades ago as one among many criteria that scientists should consider when choosing experimental designs. "*External validity* asks the question of *generalizability:* To what populations, settings, treatment variables, and measurement variables can this effect be generalized?" (Campbell and Stanley 1967, p. 5, quoted in Mook 1983, p. 379). In a lively discussion of the issue of external validity, Mook (1983) challenged the assumption that external validity is actually necessary in the case of much experimental psychological research, noting that "the distinction between generality of findings and generality of theoretical conclusions underscores what seems to me the most important source of confusion in all this, which is the assumption that the purpose of collecting data in the laboratory is to *predict real-life behavior in the real world. . . .* When it is, then the problem of [external validity] confronts us, full force" (p. 381). Mook suggests that the central distinction lies in the difference between claiming "what *can* happen, rather than what typically *does*" (p. 384). In other words, the conclusions of experimental research (that need not meet the standards of external validity) should be about a theory and not about a population. This is not to say that laboratory results cannot be generalized to the real world. Rather, we must ask how well the finding describes the phenomenon.

Artificial versus real events.   The issue of generalizability is critical when the findings of experimental laboratory studies of memory are extended to provide explanations of or predictions about clinical phenomena. In such cases, questions of the generalizability of manipulations, settings, measures, and subjects require attention. Many clinical and some experimental researchers have voiced substantial reservations about the application of findings from the experimental study of the effects of negative mood/arousal on memory to explicating real-world phenomena, such as eyewitness testimony in the forensic domain (Yuille and Cutshall 1986) or posttraumatic memory in the clinical domain (Olio and Cornell 1994; Tromp et al. 1995; van der Kolk and Fisler 1995). They note that laboratory studies use artificial events (e.g., slide, video, or staged incidents), and subjects know this. Consequently, experimental settings and manipulations may lack many of the natural elements of an emotion-evoking experience such as immediacy, surprise, and personal consequence. In addition, the success of the manipulation in evoking a degree of negative emotion or arousal comparable to real-world situations is questionable. This may be unavoidable because it would be as unethical for cognitive researchers to expose subjects to truly traumatizing manipulations as it would be for clinical researchers to randomly assign children to abusive parents. Nevertheless, the generalizability of research findings is predicated on the assumption that the manipulation models the real-world event.

Laboratory events are also not personally relevant autobiographical events in which subjects are active participants. Consequently, generalizing findings based on laboratory events requires the assumption that the same basic processing characteristics apply across differing situations. Moreover, laboratory studies of memory typically involve recall and recognition assessment hours to days later, whereas forensic settings may require that memory be assessed days to years after the event in question occurred and clinical situations may include a time frame of decades. These issues are central to the determination of whether experimental findings may be appropriately generalized to explain and predict phenomena beyond the confines of the laboratory.

Using nonclinical subjects.   Another condition of external validity—the generalizability of the findings from one's sample to the population of interest—is particularly nettlesome in discussions of trauma and memory. A large number, perhaps the majority, of experimental cognitive psychology studies use college students as subjects. Yuille and Cutshall (1986) reported that, from 1974 to 1982, 92% of research articles pertaining to eyewitness testimony used college students exclusively. Therefore, legitimate questions of generalizability center on whether findings with respect to this young, accomplished, and well-educated sample can be assumed to apply to the general population. Presumably, the assumption of experimental psychologists, as evidenced by their faithful commitment to this pool of subjects, is that they can. Taking a cue from Mook (1983), it would seem that this confidence rests on the fact that experimentalists seek to describe and understand basic processes, to understand "what can happen."

Obviously, the issue of generalizability of experimental findings derived from studies of college students to clinical populations is more complicated still. The generalization here is from a select group of nonclinical subjects to a select group of subjects with psychiatric disturbances that are the target of the generalization (e.g., depression, posttraumatic reactions, dissociation) and that may be associated with other characteristics that could vary between clinical and nonclinical populations (e.g., level of functioning, motivation). To support such a generalization, one must assume that the variable under study lies on a psychological continuum that spans these populations. In other words, the processes in pathological conditions are fundamentally the same as those in nonpathological conditions—the difference is quantitative rather than qualitative. This critical assumption has not gone entirely unnoticed or unquestioned in the experimental mood and memory research that seeks generalization to clinical depression. Commentators have cautioned about generalizing from laboratory-induced depressed mood or naturally occurring nonpathological dysphoric affect to clinical depression (e.g., Ingram 1989).

This issue comes into particularly sharp focus, we believe, in discussions of the findings of experimental study of memories for events associated with negative affect/high arousal. If we adhere to the experimental findings and Christianson's (1992) conclusions from his extensive review of this literature, then we would conclude that high-stress events seem to be better remembered than low-stress events, especially in memory of the central details. However, a survey of 63 experts in eyewitness psychology found a different opinion (Kassin et al. 1989). Specifically, almost 80% of these experts agreed with a statement that the available evidence suggested that very high levels of stress impair the accuracy of eyewitness testimony, and most of them believed that nonviolent acts were better remembered than violent ones. Christianson (1992) suggested that this apparent expert consensus may be due to experts' selective attention to several widely cited eyewitness studies (those considered most relevant to forensic concerns) that failed to disambiguate reporting of central and peripheral details or found impairment only in recall of peripheral material. On the other hand, expert opinion is not inconsistent with clinical descriptions of those who have endured profound traumatic experiences and subsequently developed posttraumatic symptomatology—a different population from the one typically used in cognitive research.

Stress versus traumatic stress.   One of the major limitations to the applicability of the experimental literature to the clinical issue of traumatic memories has been the failure to consistently examine the memory characteristics of populations that have been *significantly* traumatized rather than just emotionally perturbed or upset. In the studies described earlier in this chapter, "traumatic events" are variously defined to include anything from watching a stranger being injured in a series of slides, to hearing about a presidential assassination, to actually being the victim of a violent assault. Obviously, for virtually everyone, the first two events are not equivalent to the third in their personal relevance or significance, immediacy, perceptual experience, emotion-evoking potential, or personal consequences. It seems reasonable, therefore, to consider that they may not be equivalent in their memorability or perhaps even in the kind of processing they evoke.

Even to generalize findings regarding personal memories of events that college students and others label as traumatic to those of individuals who have experienced events that would fulfill Criterion A of the DSM-IV (American Psychiatric Association 1994) diagnosis of posttraumatic stress disorder (PTSD)[1] assumes a dose-response relationship between negative emotional experience and memory that begs the question.[2] This is particularly problematic because about one-quarter of this latter group are estimated to go on to develop PTSD symptomatology (Green 1994), which may include significant and diagnostic *disturbances* in memory, such as flashbacks and/or amnesia for some or all of the traumatic event.

This unexamined factor—the differing prevalences of PTSD symptoms in the populations in different studies—may account for some of the discrepant findings in the eyewitness literature. Some studies have reported that witnesses to a murder, even those reporting the highest amount of stress, were highly accurate in their reports (the memories were "detailed, accurate and persistent") when interviewed soon after the event and when reinterviewed 4–5 months later (Yuille and Cutshall 1986, p. 181) and that victims of a post office robbery (i.e., the teller facing the gun) were significantly more accurate than bystanders who witnessed the event (Christianson and Hubinette 1993). However, other studies have found decrements in memory for traumatic experiences. For example, in a recent report examining characteristics of intensely pleasant, intensely unpleasant (nonrape), and rape memories, Tromp and her colleagues (1995) found that although memories of rape were more affectively negative than the other reported unpleasant memories, they were actually less clear and vivid, were less well remembered, had less meaningful order, and were less thought and talked about. Similarly, in a study of victims of violent crimes, Kuehn (1974) found that victims of more serious crimes (e.g., rape or assault) provided less rich descriptions of the crime to the police than victims of less serious crimes (e.g., robberies), and injured victims provided less information than uninjured victims regardless of the type of crime.

To reconcile these disparate findings, it seems reasonable to speculate that victims of more serious or injurious crimes would be more likely

---

[1] Criterion A in the DSM-IV diagnosis of PTSD requires that "the person has been exposed to a traumatic event in which both of the following were present: (1) the person experienced, witnessed, or was confronted with an event or events that involved actual or threatened death or serious injury, or a threat to the physical integrity of self or others," and "(2) the person's response involved intense fear, helplessness, or horror" (American Psychiatric Association 1994, pp. 427–428).

[2] Interestingly, a dose-response relationship has been established between physical proximity to a traumatic event and the development and severity of PTSD symptoms (Mueser and Butler 1987; Pynoos et al. 1987).

to have posttraumatic symptoms than victims of less serious or injurious crimes or than witnesses to crimes.[3] In other words, emotional arousal may enhance memory but only up to a point; after that point, negative emotion or high arousal (or their combination) may have a qualitatively different, disorganizing effect on memory function, and posttraumatic symptomatology may represent its residue. This is a view that the descriptive clinical literature has long and widely recorded (e.g., Brett and Ostroff 1985; Harvey and Herman 1994; Horowitz 1986; Janet 1889, 1909b, cited in van der Kolk and van der Hart 1991; Janet 1907; D. Spiegel and Cardeña 1991; van der Kolk and Fisler 1995; van der Kolk and van der Hart 1989, 1991).

Two central aspects of memory disturbance in posttraumatic conditions are not reflected in the empirical cognitive literature descriptions of memory for emotional events. These aspects reflect the clinical observation that, with respect to trauma, patients seem to remember either too much (intrusion symptoms) or too little (avoidance symptoms, specifically amnesia) (Horowitz 1986; van der Kolk and van der Hart 1991). We briefly examine these aspects in turn.

Effects of Negative Affect on Recall: Clinical Data

Memory disturbance in posttraumatic conditions: intrusion symptoms. The questions posed above about the applicability of laboratory findings regarding normal memory function to clinically significant traumatic memories are underscored when the features of posttraumatic memory are described. van der Kolk and van der Hart (1989, 1991; Janet 1889, 1919/1925, cited in van der Kolk and van der Hart 1991; Janet 1907; van der Kolk and Fisler 1995) proposed that the "traumatic memories" described in clinical populations as intrusion symptoms are qualitatively different from normal narrative memory and include sensory, affective, and motoric reliving experiences, flashbacks, nightmares, and behavioral reenactments. They appear to represent a distinct departure from normal memory processing.

The unbidden, vivid, and absorbing experience of a flashback or reliving of the traumatic event is one of the most profoundly disturbing intrusion symptoms in posttraumatic reactions. During these episodes, which may last from a few seconds to several hours, the traumatic event is not just remembered but reexperienced in the moment. This event presumably reflects a state of absorption into the content or fragment of a memory or belief and its attendant affect that is so profound that

---

[3]An alternative explanation of these particular findings could be that victims may be focusing their attention on their pain or injuries and consequently not encoding other characteristics of the event (G. Bower, personal communication, April 1996).

the current environment is largely ignored and the individual temporarily does not distinguish memory from present experience (Butler et al. 1996; Maldonado and Spiegel 1994). Such flashbacks, or relivings of the event, may be triggered by environmental stimuli reminiscent of the trauma and may occur even decades after the original event (Brockway 1988). Traumatic memories also may be experienced as distressing nightmares, either identical in experience to waking flashbacks or as more regular dreams intermixing traumatic and other material (van der Kolk and Fisler 1995). Sometimes such dreams can only be inferred from the patient's reports of having disturbing dreams for which he or she remembers few specifics or from accounts of his or her bed partner who witnessed the patient's utterances, screams, and movements (Maldonado and Spiegel 1994). Studies of posttraumatic nightmares indicate that the traumatic scenes may be repeated without modification, even for extended periods (e.g., 15 years) (van der Kolk et al. 1984).

Freud (1914/1958) observed that for some traumatized patients the memory of the event is experienced in the form of a motoric behavioral reenactment of the actions originally taken in the face of trauma. This reenactment "reproduces [the experience] not as a memory but as an action: he repeats it, without knowing, of course, that he is repeating, and in the end, we understand that this is his way of remembering" (quoted in van der Kolk and van der Hart 1991, p. 436). Terr (1988) described a related phenomenon, which she termed *behavioral memories,* in 18 of 20 children she studied who had experienced psychic trauma before age 5 years. She noted that for more than three-quarters of the children, their play, fears, or personality changes "strikingly mirrored" (p. 98) what had been documented about their histories.[4] Terr also observed that these behavioral memories were quite accurate and true to the events that stimulated them regardless of whether the trauma had occurred before or after language acquisition.

Differences in encoding, storage, and retrieval of traumatic memories. To explain these distressing and bizarre posttraumatic symptoms, investigators have proposed that some experiences may be so overwhelming that they cannot be integrated into existing normal mental frameworks and consequently are encoded differently (D. Spiegel 1984, 1986; van der Hart and Spiegel 1993; van der Kolk and Fisler 1995; van der Kolk and van der Hart 1991). Siegel (1995) enumerated the following factors that may be present in traumatic experiences and may influence the differential memory processing of these events:

---

[4]Note, however, that the rater was not blind in this study, thus a confirmation bias may have increased the likelihood of her noting a correspondence between the children's behaviors and the documentation of their traumatic experiences.

- The overwhelming emotions and extreme stress or physical pain during the event may impede processing of perceptual inputs.
- If the event is novel in the individual's experience, it may also overwhelm perceptual attention processes and/or deviate from preestablished schemata or mental models, thereby limiting possible encoding.
- Cognitive adaptations (such as perceptual avoidance, divided attention, escape fantasy, somatic numbing), the meaning of the event (loss, betrayal, abandonment), and the social context in which it occurs may all disrupt the processing necessary for consolidation of normal long-term memory.

Clearly, most of these features are absent (for ethical reasons) in laboratory studies of emotion and memory.

Janet (1889, 1907, 1919/1925, described in van der Kolk and van der Hart 1989, 1991) first proposed that traumatic memories represent the intrusive return of unassimilated material in fragmentary sensory, affective, and motoric form. van der Kolk and van der Hart (1991), in summarizing Janet's views, noted

> that the ease with which current experience is integrated into existing mental structures depends on the subjective assessment of what is happening; familiar and expectable experiences are automatically assimilated without much conscious awareness of details of the particulars, while frightening or novel experiences may not easily fit into existing cognitive schemes and be remembered with particular vividness, or totally resist integration. Under extreme conditions, existing meaning schemes may be entirely unable to accommodate frightening experiences, which causes the "memory" of these experiences to be stored differently, and not be available for retrieval under ordinary conditions: it becomes dissociated from conscious awareness and voluntary control. . . . When that occurs, fragments of these unintegrated experiences may later manifest recollections or behavioral reenactments. (p. 427)

van der Kolk (1987) also observed that people who are exposed to significant trauma experience a "speechless terror," and organization of the experience, at least initially, is without semantic representation. "The experience cannot be organized on a linguistic level and this failure to arrange the memory into words and symbols leaves it to be organized on a somatosensory or iconic level: as somatic sensations, behavioral reenactments, nightmares, and flashbacks" (van der Kolk and van der Hart 1991, p. 443). Schacter (1987; see also Siegel 1995) has suggested that traumatic memories, such as those that Janet described, may represent implicit memories of the trauma.

To remedy the intrusion of "the unassimilated scraps of overwhelming experiences" (p. 447) that present as traumatic memories, van der

Kolk and van der Hart (1991) suggested that these experiences need to be integrated with existing mental structures and transformed into narrative language. van der Kolk and Ducey (1989, p. 271) concluded that "a sudden and passively endured trauma is relived repeatedly, until a person learns to remember simultaneously the affect and cognition associated with the trauma through access to language."

Based on Janet's observations and their own, van der Kolk and colleagues (van der Kolk and Fisler 1995, see Table 2, p. 521; van der Kolk and van der Hart 1991) have enumerated four features that distinguish traumatic (intrusive) memories and normal narrative memories:

1. Traumatic memories are composed of images, sensations, and affective and behavioral states, whereas narrative memory is semantic and symbolic and may be conveyed verbally.
2. Traumatic memories are inflexible and invariant over time, whereas narrative memories serve social and adaptive functions.
3. Traumatic memories cannot be evoked at will but are automatically elicited under specific circumstances reminiscent of the original event; once one element of the memory is stimulated, the retrieval floodgates open, and the other elements are recalled (reexperienced). In contrast, narrative memories are generally accessible without triggers, and they do not bring with them an irrepressible constellation of associated affective, somatic, and motoric experiences.
4. Traumatic memories, which effectively reconstitute some or all of the trauma through behavioral reenactment or intrapsychic replay, take time to "remember," whereas narrative memories are verbal distillations that may be condensed or expanded on social demands.

A fascinating recent exploratory study further examined the differences between intrusive memories for traumatic events and nontraumatic memories. In this study, van der Kolk and Fisler (1995) recruited and assessed 46 nonclinical adults "who were haunted by memories of terrible life experiences" (p. 514). All subjects' symptoms met DSM-III-R (American Psychiatric Association 1987) criteria for PTSD. The subjects were interviewed to assess a variety of characteristics of their traumatic memories and then were asked the same questions about an intense, nontraumatic experience of their choice (e.g., birthdays, graduations, weddings, births of children). Of the subjects whose traumatic memories were of childhood events (more than 75% of the sample), 42% had endured significant or total amnesia for the experience at some time in their lives. More than 75% of the entire sample reported nightmares, some of which were identical to their flashbacks and others that were dreams incorporating non-trauma-related material or illogical combinations of material. *All* subjects claimed that they initially "remembered" the traumatic event as somatosensory flashback experiences, presenting in a variety of somatosensory modalities and emotions, rather than in coherent narrative form. These traumatic memories were reported to develop over time, involving more and more modalities, and ultimately were constructed into a narrative by the subject (although 11% of the sample were still unable to convey a coherent narrative of the event—all of these subjects had endured childhood traumas). The authors concluded that "traumatic 'memories,' per se, consist of emotional and sensory states, with little verbal representation" (p. 520). Interestingly, none of the significant *nontraumatic* memories were experienced as dreams, flashbacks, or somatosensory relivings; none were associated with amnesic periods; none had a photographic quality; none were reexperienced as vivid memories after environmental triggers; and in no case did subjects attempt to suppress them. van der Kolk and Fisler (1995, p. 520; see also Siegel 1995; van der Kolk and Ducey 1989) concluded that "traumatic experiences in people with PTSD are initially imprinted as sensations or feeling states that are not immediately transcribed into personal narratives. This failure to process information on a symbolic level following trauma is at the very core of the pathology of PTSD."

In the preceding section, we describe the intrusive traumatic memory symptoms of flashbacks, nightmares, and behavioral reenactments that characterize some posttraumatic conditions. These clinically significant traumatic memories represent what appears to involve a breakdown or qualitative shift in processing that occurs in the face of extreme affect rather than a quantitative enhancement of memory such as the experimental literature would suggest. These traumatic memories are unique in that they are represented in nonverbal modalities, they are accompanied by intense affect, and their retrieval is outside of conscious control. In the next section, we discuss the most severe posttraumatic memory disturbance—another memory presentation that is not accounted for in the experimental literature—amnesia.

Memory disturbance in posttraumatic conditions: traumatic amnesia. Although amnesia for childhood sexual abuse is currently an issue of much debate (e.g., Loftus 1993; Loftus and Ketcham 1994; Ofshe and Singer 1994; Ofshe and Watters 1994), cases of amnesia after traumatic or highly emotional events have been widely reported in relation to many different traumatic experiences, such as natural disasters and accidents (e.g., van der Kolk and Kadish 1987; Wilkinson 1983), and seem to be especially common after physical or psychological assaults, such as combat (e.g., Grinker and Spiegel 1945; Kardiner 1941; Kardiner and Spiegel 1947), concentration camp experiences (Jaffe 1968), and torture (Goldfield et al. 1988).

In the last two decades, the documentation of child sexual abuse has increased greatly (e.g., Finkelhor et al. 1990; Russell 1983; Wyatt 1985); along with this, a number of studies of adult survivors who claim periods of not remembering some or all of their abuse history at some time in their lives have been published. Among these are reports of partial to complete traumatic amnesia among 59%–64% of help-seeking childhood sexual abuse survivors (Albach 1993, 1995, reported in Bowman, in press a; Briere and Conte 1993; Herman and Schatzow 1987), 34%–40% of therapists with childhood sexual abuse histories (Feldman-Summers and Pope 1994; Polusny and Follette 1996), and 31%–44% of samples of adult survivors who were not therapists or seeking treatment for sexual abuse (Elliot and Briere 1995, community sample; Elliot and Fox 1994, college students; Loftus et al. 1994b, substance abuse patients; van der Kolk and Fisler 1995, subjects recruited because of traumatic memories).

The most compelling evidence to date of traumatic amnesia for childhood sexual abuse has been presented by Williams (1994a, 1995; see also Williams and Banyard, Chapter 9, in this volume). In this study, Williams (1994a) contacted women with established histories of childhood sexual abuse documented in emergency room records of a major city hospital during the early 1970s. Subjects were asked detailed questions about their childhood and life experiences, including childhood experiences with sex. The results of these interviews were striking: 38% of these women did not report the abuse that had been recorded 17 years earlier nor did they report any sexual abuse by the same perpetrator (this includes 12% of the entire sample who reported no abuse at all) (Williams 1994a). If the analysis was conservatively restricted to only those subjects with recorded medical evidence of genital trauma and whose accounts were rated as most credible (in the 1970s), 52% did not remember the sexual abuse. Of the women who did remember the abuse, 16% (10% of the entire sample) reported that there was a time when they did not remember the abuse (Williams 1995).

The Williams study (1994a) also has implications for the levels of reporting in the other studies described above. In each of those, the subjects had to remember the abuse to be able to report that they had at some point forgotten it. The findings of the Williams study suggest that some women who do not remember childhood sexual abuse may well have endured it and currently have traumatic amnesia for the experience. This group, however small or large it might be, is not represented in the rates of amnesia reported in most studies, suggesting that, as startling as prevalences reported above may be, they are likely to be underestimates of the true prevalence of traumatic amnesia among childhood sexual abuse survivors. Because no comparison groups were used in these studies, it is impossible to determine the extent to which the findings deviate from normal forgetting of non-abuse-related childhood events.

There is also evidence for more generalized memory impairment in some traumatized individuals. In an unpublished study (Vardi, cited in D. Brown 1995), memory performance was compared among women who had a history of incest, women who were raped as adults, and women who had no history of sexual molestation. The results indicated that both molested groups had acute PTSD symptoms, but only the incest survivors had chronic PTSD symptoms and significant impairments in personal autobiographical memory nonspecific to the abuse, such as remembering names of teachers, schools attended, and significant public events. These impairments occurred especially for the period of life associated with the incest—a finding reminiscent of the central versus peripheral detail recall evidence. Additionally, Bremner et al. (1993) found that patients with combat-related PTSD had deficits in short-term memory; these deficits may be related to the lower hippocampal volume also found in this population (Bremner et al. 1995b).

In summary, the experimental psychological literature on emotion/stress and memory seems to be correct up to a point: In general, memory for the central details and overall theme of a traumatic event may be enhanced by the increased negative affect associated with an event, whereas memory for peripheral or contextual information may be diminished. Christianson (1992) rejected the notion of a Yerkes-Dodson (1908) inverted U relationship between increasing stress and memory function, because the conclusions of his review did not support it (i.e., he did not find the descending arm of the association). It appears, however, that his literature survey was generally limited to nonclinical samples, and consequently, his conclusions describe a rather truncated portion of the possible sample of traumatizing experiences and traumatized individuals.

The clinical literature, on the other hand, suggests that with respect to individuals with posttraumatic conditions, the quantitative association (of increasing stress and improved retention/recall) may be replaced by a qualitatively different one in which intense fear, helplessness, or horror overwhelms the individual and exerts a destabilizing effect on the process of memory consolidation and/or accessibility (Horowitz 1986; van der Kolk and van der Hart 1991). Individuals who have experienced significant trauma, especially those with PTSD symptomatology, seem to represent a different population, exhibiting a contrasting response, in what are likely incomparable conditions, when compared with subjects in experimental studies of emotional arousal and memory. We concur with Harvey and Herman's (1994) somewhat understated conclusion that "future research into the nature of traumatic memory should be informed by clinical observation" (p. 295).

Some cognitive psychologists have argued that memory failure in survivors of childhood sexual abuse can be explained by theories of normal forgetting and that no special process need be inferred. We consider these arguments next.

Explanations for Traumatic Amnesia

Some cognitive psychologists (Bower 1990; Loftus 1993; Loftus et al. 1994a) have suggested that the concepts of repression or dissociation do not need to be invoked to explain the findings of memory inaccessibility among trauma victims. Rather, they suggest that ordinary forgetting (Loftus 1993; Loftus et al. 1994a), motivated forgetting (Bower 1990), or inadequate retrieval cues (Bower 1990) may account for the phenomenon.

Ordinary forgetting and motivated forgetting. Put simply, the "ordinary forgetting" explanation suggests that a survivor may just forget that she or he was repeatedly and violently molested over the course of years by her or his father. In support of this view, Loftus (1993) noted that people routinely forget important events, such as car accidents and hospitalizations. Bower (1990; see also Koutstaal and Schacter, Chapter 8, in this volume) adds the element of motivation to his analysis, thereby accommodating the aversive nature of the experience. He suggests that motivated nonlearning (through lack of attention, nonrehearsal, or automatized avoidance of unpleasant cognitions) or motivated overwriting of memories (learning new associations) may interfere with encoding or storage and thus make some memories difficult to retrieve. As Koutstaal and Schacter (Chapter 8 in this volume) point out, a motivated forgetting explanation of traumatic amnesia is consistent with the anecdotal descriptions of attempting to "block out" memories reported by some of the childhood sexual abuse survivors in the Williams study (1995). However, this hypothesis has no direct experimental support. Findings to date suggest that the more traumatizing the event (e.g., presence of PTSD in those who experienced it), the less successful attempts may be not to remember or think of it (for a discussion, see Koutstaal and Schacter, Chapter 8, in this volume). In addition, as Bower (1990) concedes, this model does not specify the conditions under which these types of mechanisms would come into operation and consequently does not explain why some unpleasant memories are (too) well recalled, whereas others are seemingly unretrievable. (It can be said that the repression and dissociation models of traumatic amnesia also fail to specify the conditions that would predict when these defense mechanisms would operate.)

Retrieval cue insufficiency. Bower (1990) suggested that inadequate retrieval cues probably contribute most to forgetting. Memory retrieval depends largely on the amount and appropriateness of the information contained in the cue (Bower 1990, 1991; Kihlstrom 1994). The adequacy of a cue also depends on the characteristics of the encoding (Tulving and Thompson 1973) and storage of that memory—if it has few or weakened associations, as might be the case with events that elicit motivated nonlearning or overwriting, then more will be required of the cue for successful retrieval. In simple terms, the cue insufficiency argument (Bower 1990) implies then that asking a woman if she had ever been molested may not be an adequate retrieval cue to elicit the memory that her father sexually molested her when she was a child. In addition, Bower (1990) suggested that there may be a motivated avoidance of certain lines of self-cues that might elicit unpleasant memories, thereby reducing the likelihood of an individual's simply coming upon such memories through a natural stream of consciousness.

Normal memory failure versus amnesia. Some of these investigators' resistance to considering or describing such memory inaccessibility as evidence of amnesia may be due to a misunderstanding of the characteristics of dissociative amnesia. For example, in a discussion of the Williams study (1994a), Loftus et al. (1994a) reject the notion of amnesia to describe the findings, stating:

> One could, of course, say that the women whom Williams studied constitute cases of complete amnesia. . . . This would mean, however, that when we forget anything, it is an example of complete amnesia for that thing. It dilutes the meaning of the term "amnesia," which has often been reserved for discussing a pathological sort of forgetting. It is rather similar to using the word "assassination" to describe the squashing of a bug. Given the new broad-ranging definition of amnesia, how would we describe what happens to the person who goes into the supermarket specifically to get aspirin and leaves 10 minutes later with a Snickers bar, a magazine, a box of Pop-Tarts, and no aspirin? Is this amnesia, or is it simply a case of forgetting? (p. 1178)

We find this logic difficult to follow and the analogies rather perverse. Moreover, the argument ignores the characteristics that define "pathological forgetting" (i.e., dissociative amnesia) outlined below, and it belittles the significance of the event and of the forgetting (see also Williams 1994b). Five central features of dissociative amnesia (as an isolated condition or as part of another dissociative disorder) should be considered (American Psychiatric Association 1994; Butler et al. 1996):

1. It involves the inability to recall important personal information.
2. The memory loss is "too extensive to be explained by normal forgetfulness" (American Psychiatric Association 1994, p. 481).
3. The unretrievable content is "usually of a traumatic or stressful nature" (American Psychiatric Association 1994, p. 481).

4. The amnesia is functional rather than organic and, therefore, potentially reversible (i.e., the information is inaccessible rather than lost, as would be the case if it had never been encoded or was somehow erased).
5. The information may still exert an influence on cognitive function, even though it is inaccessible to consciousness—it is out of sight but not out of mind (as is suggested by the heightened reactivity and other posttraumatic symptoms that bring some amnesic survivors of childhood sexual abuse into treatment).

All of these features may be identified in many adults who are amnesic for their histories of childhood sexual abuse. Consequently, although in this chapter we have used the term *traumatic amnesia* to describe extensive forgetting of childhood sexual abuse, it may be that many of these individuals would have symptoms that meet criteria for a formal DSM-IV diagnosis of dissociative amnesia.

Also, note that traumatic amnesia among adult survivors of childhood sexual abuse is not randomly distributed, as might be consistent with an ordinary forgetting or cue insufficiency explanation. Instead, in most studies in which amnesia has been examined, it is associated with factors that would presumably make the event more memorable, such as more violent or more chronic abuse (Briere and Conte 1993; Herman and Schatzow 1987), or factors that would conceivably have a greater effect on the child's developing identity and life experience, such as being younger at the time of the abuse and being molested by someone he or she knew, especially a family member (Briere and Conte 1993; Feldman-Summers and Pope 1994; Herman and Schatzow 1987; Williams 1994a, 1995). In other words, the greater the predictable psychological or developmental effect, the more likely the life experience will be forgotten by these individuals—clearly, this is contrary to what might be predicted from normal processes of memory failure, and it is inconsistent with the extensive cognitive literature on increased memorability of emotional events in nonclinical subjects (Christianson 1992).

Of course, the preceding observation assumes that sexual molestation in childhood is a significant, often life-altering, experience for most people. And that certainly seems to be what many adult survivors report—both those who continuously remember their abuse histories and those who recover memories as adults—particularly those who seek treatment for its ongoing effects on their lives. Childhood sexual abuse is associated with higher rates of many adult psychopathological sequelae, including depression, sexual dysfunction, substance abuse, interpersonal difficulties, revictimization, and PTSD (reviewed in Beitchman et al. 1992; Polusny and Follette 1995; Rowan and Foy 1993; Rowan et al. 1994) in both clinical and nonclinical samples. Some investigators debate, however, whether a distinct post–sexual abuse syndrome exists (Beitchman et al. 1992; cf. Finkelhor 1988), and others even question the basic claim of child sexual abuse as an etiological factor in adult psychiatric disorders, because studies reporting such associations are inadequately controlled (Pope and Hudson 1995).

Repetition and memory. The association between chronic abuse and amnesia for the event also raises another issue that we believe challenges even the motivated forgetting explanation—that is, one of rehearsal. Bower's (1990) description of motivated forgetting would seem most applicable in cases of memories for isolated events, because it depends on the limitation or relative weakening of associations. It would seem to be hard pressed, however, to accommodate the memory effects of repeated abuse experiences, which may be viewed as rehearsals of the event in experience and memory (P. Jasiukaitis, personal communication, April 1996).

To reiterate the general point, it would seem that "single blow" traumas (Terr 1991) should be the events most likely to be forgotten because they are single events and presumably, therefore, less existentially meaningful and less likely to prompt the development of a memory category or cognitive schema for such an episode, they would not fit into preexisting schemata, and their rehearsal could be avoided or minimized. Repeated traumatic events (such as chronic childhood sexual abuse occurring for years), on the other hand, would represent unavoidable rehearsals of the experience and associated memories. They would accumulate as a store of autobiographical memories with elaborate associations, and consequently, they would be more likely to result in changes in general knowledge about the self and the world, in self-concept, and in schemata for the perpetrator (if he or she is known to the victim) and others perceived as being involved (e.g., denying family members) or for particular events (e.g., going to bed at night). However, the opposite often appears to be the case—the more chronic is the abuse (as well as other factors described previously), the more likely is the development of memory disturbances such as traumatic amnesia (Briere and Conte 1993; Herman and Schatzow 1987; Terr 1991).

Based on these considerations, the ordinary forgetting, motivated forgetting, or cue insufficiency arguments do not seem to offer reasonable alternative explanations for not remembering that one was sexually molested as a child or adolescent. It does seem reasonable, however, to suggest that events that might be expected to change one's life or that would change it if one knew of them would not *ordinarily* be forgotten or very difficult to retrieve and that if such information is inaccessible, then some cognitive processes are not, in fact, functioning normally.

›vered Memory

₂ preceding sections, we discussed the conflicting experimental
:linical views regarding the effects of strong negative affect on
memory and some of the possible reasons for the inaccessibility of
memories of childhood sexual abuse. An even more contentious debate
has been prompted by cognitive research into memory alteration and
implantation. In the following section, we review some of this literature
and then discuss what we believe are its limitations, urging caution in
generalizing from it to account for the clinical phenomenon of recovered memories.

Suggestion Effects: The Alteration of
Memory With Postevent Information

A considerable body of empirical literature documents that memories
for events may be altered in a variety of ways in experimental settings;
this family of effects is commonly described as the *misinformation effect*
(Garry et al. 1994). The misinformation effect generally refers to the
finding that subjects who are misled about witnessed events may incorporate inaccurate postevent information into their accounts of those
events (Garry and Loftus 1994). Another, more recent, misinformation
effect is one in which wholly new memories may be implanted through
suggestion. We briefly discuss several ways in which extant memories
may be altered and new memories introduced (adapted, in part, from
Garry and Loftus 1994; Garry et al. 1994).

The influence of leading questions on subject responses.   Loftus and
Palmer (1974) found that when subjects were shown films of car accidents, the wording of the postviewing questioning could influence
subjects' answers about the event. For example, subjects were more
likely to report greater speeds for the moving cars they had seen if they
were asked how fast the cars were going when they *smashed* into each
other than if they were asked how fast the cars were going when they
hit each other. Subjects in the former condition were also more likely
to report seeing broken glass at the scene (32% for "smashed" subjects
vs. 14% for "hit" subjects—a difference of 18%), even though none was
shown, suggesting an alteration of the memory representation of the
event.

Interestingly, in a study of accounts of real witnesses to a murder
(Yuille and Cutshall 1986), the vast majority (83%) of witnesses resisted
misleading information incorporated into interviews conducted 4–
5 months later. In this study, subjects were asked whether they saw "*a*
broken headlight" or "*the* broken headlight" on the perpetrator's car
(when there was no broken headlight) or whether they saw "*a* yellow

---

quarterpanel" or "*the* yellow quarterpanel" (when the off-color quar-terpanel was blue)—virtually all of them correctly reported that there was no broken headlight or yellow quarterpanel or that they had not noticed the detail.

The insertion by suggestion of items or objects into a previously ob-served scene. Misleading but plausible information embedded in questions about a viewed scene may also influence the content of sub-sequent recall. For example, Loftus (1975) found that when subjects were asked, "How fast was the white sports car going when it passed the barn while traveling along the country road?" (when no barn had been in the scene that was viewed), they were more likely than control subjects to report remembering seeing a barn when queried about it later (17% for misled subjects vs. 3% for control subjects—a difference of 14%).

The manipulation of details about an item or object that appeared in a previously observed scene. Loftus et al. (1978) showed subjects slides of an automobile-pedestrian accident scene in which a red car stopped at either a stop sign or a yield sign and then struck a pedestrian at a crosswalk. After viewing the slides, half of the subjects were asked a question in which the nature of the sign was altered (e.g., the stop sign was now a yield sign, and vice versa). When subjects were asked to identify the slide they had seen (given a forced choice), those sub-jects who had received the misleading information were less likely to choose the actual slide they had seen than subjects who had not re-ceived misleading information (41% vs. 75% were correct, respec-tively—a difference of 34%).

In a related line of misinformation research, Ceci and Bruck and their colleagues have presented a variety of evidence indicating that children are quite suggestible (i.e., susceptible to misinformation), and more so than adults (see Ceci and Bruck 1993, for a review). In a recent study, Bruck et al. (1995) examined the influence of postevent suggestions on children's reports of stressful events involving their own bodies—in this case, a visit to a pediatrician for an inoculation. These children were recontacted an average of 11 months after the inoculations and visited on four separate occasions over 2 weeks. During each of the first three visits, the children were given pain-denying or neutral feedback about their original experience of the inoculation and were also given mis-leading information or no information about the actions of the pedia-trician and of a research assistant who had been present at the time of the inoculation (e.g., who had given them the shot and who had showed them a poster). On the fourth visit, they were asked to state everything they could remember about the time they got their shot, to report everything that the research assistant and the pediatrician had done, and to rate how much the shot had hurt and how much they had cried at the time.

The results indicated that suggestion after a year's delay significantly influenced children's reports. Children receiving the pain-denying feedback reported less pain and crying than those receiving neutral feedback. Those who were misinformed were also more likely to make mistakes about who had done what during the original event. The authors suggest that although it is difficult to disambiguate whether these effects reflect a *change in how children report* their experiences (a social influence effect) or a *change in actual memory* for the events (a cognitive effect), some evidence suggested that reasoning-based inferential processes may have been at work. The addition of new information or of particular inaccuracies in the children's stories suggested they were trying to construct congruent mental scripts based on the misinformation and their own expectations about what must have happened. Note, however, that this last point does not necessarily indicate a change in what they remember, but rather it involves a construction of an explanation (i.e., what they believe) in the present that may or may not overwrite or alter the original memory.

Interestingly, this study also shows that suggestion effects on memory or its report may be bidirectional; that is, suggestion may deflate as well as inflate claims—in this case, pain-denying feedback resulted in retrospective reports of less pain. This is more analogous to a clinical situation in which a victim of abuse denies that an event happened than it is to one in which a psychotherapy patient falsely accuses a parent of abuse. The subjects in Bruck et al.'s study downplayed real, if mild, trauma.

Suggestion Effects: The Implantation of Memories

Clearly, the most relevant and controversial area of experimental research related to the clinical issue of recovered memories is whether individuals can be falsely convinced that something happened to them and come to "remember" experiencing that event. Although some anecdotal reports of false memories have been published (e.g., Piaget 1962; Pynoos and Nader 1989), Loftus and her colleagues (Loftus and Coan, unpublished data, reported in Loftus 1993; Loftus and Pickrell 1995; Loftus et al., in press) were the first to succeed in implanting memories in laboratory subjects without hypnosis. The implantation of memories is the only misinformation effect that involves the creation of new "memories" rather than the manipulation of existing ones.

The suggestion of entire episodes purportedly from the subject's past.
In what has become the paradigmatic memory implantation protocol, confederate graduate students attempt to lead an offspring or sibling

to believe that he or she was lost in a shopping mall when he or she was 5 years old by telling the subject that they themselves remembered the event and asking the subject to try to recall and describe the event on repeated occasions. Loftus and Pickrell (1995) reported that 25% of their subjects claimed to remember the false event of being lost in a shopping mall at age 5, either fully or partially, and generated additional details about the event (see also Loftus and Coan, described in Loftus 1993; Loftus and Ketcham 1994; Loftus et al., in press). Hyman and colleagues (Hyman et al. 1995; Hyman and Billings, unpublished manuscript, reported in Loftus et al., in press) also reported implanting false childhood memories in 20%–27% of college students. In their study, the memories included having a birthday party at age 5 at which a clown visited and pizza was served; staying overnight at the hospital for a high fever and earache; attending a wedding and accidentally spilling a punch bowl; and evacuating a grocery store because a sprinkler had been activated—events chosen because they were presumably more unusual than the common experience of being lost or fearing being lost in a mall as a child.

In a study of source misattribution in children, Ceci et al. (1994) were also able to implant and study false memories. In this experiment, children were instructed to identify the events they actually remembered among four actual (parent-supplied) and four fictional (experimenter-contrived) events (one positive, negative, neutral-participant, neutral-nonparticipant for each type) described to them by the investigator. For each event, the children were told that their mothers had said it had occurred, were asked to try to visualize it, and were instructed to try to recall it on 12 separate occasions approximately 1 week apart. The results indicated that children almost always remembered the actual events, and more than 40% of them reported remembering at least one fictional event by the final session. The children were *least* susceptible to assenting to negative fictional events (e.g., falling off a tricycle and getting stitches) than to any other type of fictional event. Ceci et al. (1994, p. 315) noted that this finding is consistent "with claims that abusive or threatening events may be more resistant to false suggestions than neutral ones."

Pezdek (1995) proposed that the probability of suggestively implanting a memory may depend on the extent to which the event is familiar because of experience or knowledge and whether one has script knowledge already accessible. To test this hypothesis, she modified the Loftus et al. paradigm by having confederates suggest to their siblings or relatives three memories—one true event, one false yet familiar event (being lost at the mall), and one false and unfamiliar event (receiving a rectal enema). The results confirmed the prediction: three subjects "remembered" being lost at the mall (15%) and recalled additional details of this event, but *not a single subject remembered receiving an enema.* Because prior testing with different subjects had revealed differences in expected frequency and in the amount of information contained in the average mental script for each event, the author concluded that false memories involving familiar events are more easily planted than false memories of unfamiliar events. As Pezdek observed, "because the findings of Loftus and Coan . . . are frequently applied to cases involving adults' memory for childhood sexual abuse (Loftus 1993), it is especially important to evaluate the appropriateness of this generalization. The results of the present study suggest that it should be far more difficult to plant false memories of childhood sexual abuse than false memories of being lost in a mall as a child" (pp. 19–20).

Pezdek also noted another implication of her findings: "It should be easier to implant false memories of childhood sexual abuse with people for whom childhood sexual contact with an adult was more familiar than with people for whom childhood sexual contact with an adult was less familiar" (p. 20). It is worth reiterating, however, that familiarity with a particular type of event may be acquired by means other than personal experience (e.g., through vicarious learning of the experiences of others or reading or viewing material about such an event).

In summary, several recent studies have reported that false memories for some childhood events may be implanted in up to 27% of adult subjects (Hyman and Billings, unpublished manuscript, reported in Loftus et al., in press; Hyman et al. 1995; Loftus and Pickrell 1995; Pezdek 1995); however, some preliminary evidence indicates that the memory creation may depend on the individual's familiarity with the event.

The alteration and implantation of memories with hypnosis. The alteration and implantation of memories have also been achieved during hypnotic trance states, and this fact is of particular significance to therapists who use hypnosis as a tool for memory recovery. Hypnosis is a state of highly focused attention, usually coupled with physical relaxation. It is also characterized by a tendency to dissociate information (keep it out of conscious awareness) that would ordinarily be conscious and by a heightened responsiveness to social cues or suggestibility (H. Spiegel and Spiegel 1987). The ability to experience this state, termed *hypnotizability,* is a stable and measurable trait (Hilgard 1965; H. Spiegel and Spiegel 1987). Hypnotizability is as consistent over a 25-year interval in adulthood as is intelligence, with test-retest correlations in the range of .7 (Piccione et al. 1989). Hypnotizability is highest in late childhood and declines gradually throughout adulthood (Morgan and Hilgard 1973). This age difference is important, because it means that children are likely to be more vulnerable to suggestive influence.

Hypnotic phenomena may occur without a formal induction (H. Spiegel and Spiegel 1987); consequently, children and others could respond suggestively either to traumatic events or to suggestive influence about them (e.g., "it did not happen, it wasn't so bad"). Because the focus of attention is narrowed in hypnosis (Tellegen 1981; Tellegen and Atkinson 1974), hypnotized individuals are more likely than others to incorporate a central idea or image rather than judge it. They would thus seem to be at elevated risk for incorporating a deliberate or unwitting suggestion into their memory reports. Indeed, Laurence et al. (1986) noted that Janet used hypnosis explicitly to alter some of a patient's memories so that the events contained in them were no longer as traumatic (see also van der Kolk and van der Hart 1989; for descriptions, see Ellenberger 1970, pp. 361–364).

Laurence and Perry (1983) experimentally demonstrated that memories for fictitious events may be created with hypnosis. In this study, 27 hypnotized subjects were age regressed to a night during the previous week in which they reported sleeping soundly. The investigators then subtly suggested, through questioning, that these now "sleeping" subjects had heard a noise. While hypnotized, almost two-thirds of subjects reported that they had indeed heard a noise. After termination of the trance state, almost half of all subjects still believed that they had heard the noise that night. Even after being told that the noise had been suggested by the hypnotist and was not in fact real, more than one-fifth of subjects retained their belief. It should be noted that the investigators' efficacy in implanting the memory was likely enhanced by the fact that it was suggested to have occurred when the subjects were asleep; that is, there was no competition from a real memory, which might have made the implanted one less plausible.

In a recent replication of this study, Lynn et al. (1994) compared responses of highly hypnotizable subjects with simulating low hypnotizable subjects. The authors concluded that because "the simulating subjects were able to role-play the responses of the hypnotized subjects successfully . . . this raises the possibility that the memory reports of hypnotic subjects may reflect their response to situational demands or reporting biases rather than actual memory changes" (p. 124).

Spanos and his colleagues (reviewed in Spanos et al. 1994) have examined the ways in which some subjects construct elaborate and complex fantasies of past-life experiences, UFO alien contact/abduction, and childhood ritual satanic abuse that they believe to be memories. Their investigations have focused on these (usually hypnotically created) pseudomemories as a means to study the processes involved in the development of what Spanos believes is an analogous condition— dissociative identity disorder (formerly known as multiple personality disorder; see also Ganaway 1989). Spanos contends that all these conditions are learned and socially constructed. Evidence for this comes from findings that characteristics of these "memories" are influenced by expectations transmitted by the experimenter. For example, in one study of "past-life regression" (Spanos et al. 1991), half of the subjects were told, before the regression, that children in earlier historical periods had frequently been abused. During the regression, these subjects reported significantly higher rates of abuse in their past-life identities than subjects not receiving this information. On termination of the hypnotic regression procedure, some subjects still reported believing that their experiences were actual memories of reincarnations.

The above studies notwithstanding, in reviewing the literature on pseudomemories and hypnotic suggestibility, D. Brown (1995, p. 6) concluded that "it is quite clear that hypnotizability, not a formal hypnotic induction, contributes significantly to PM [pseudomemory] production; PM rates are about the same in high-hypnotizable subjects, whether or not formal hypnotic procedures or waking instructions are used." D. Brown proposed that pseudomemory production in hypnosis is best understood as an interaction of hypnotizability and social influence and that therapists should carefully assess the risk factors for pseudomemory production in their patients, especially if they have posttraumatic stress symptoms without an identifiable stressor and with limited memories (see also Bowman, in press b).

It is important to recognize that hypnotic phenomena, including memory distortion, can occur even in the absence of a formal induction, especially among highly hypnotizable individuals (D. Spiegel 1995). Indeed, the structure of the hypnotic state, with its narrowing of focal attention, dissociation, and heightened responsiveness to social cues, shares many features with the acute dissociative state seen during and immediately after trauma (Bremner et al. 1995a; Koopman et al. 1994; Marmar et al. 1994; D. Spiegel and Cardeña 1991; for a review, see Butler et al. 1996). Therefore, it is logical that hypnotizable individuals may have spontaneously entered hypnotic-like states during traumatic experiences and, thus, be more prone to remembering them in a subsequent state of formal hypnosis. By the same token, the structure of the experience of entering a hypnotic state may elicit traumatic schemata independent of any specific content. Thus, vulnerability to the implantation of pseudomemories is higher among highly hypnotizable individuals, especially during hypnosis, because the mental state is similar in traumatic and hypnotic situations. Similarly, receptivity to the retrieval of veridical memories may also be increased because of the similarity of mental states. Consequently, hypnotized individuals may be more likely to report both suggested and veridical traumatic memories.

In short, there is mounting evidence that suggestion may cause some individuals to report false memories of past events with and without the use of hypnosis. The relative contributions of actual cognitive changes versus social conformity effects in these events have yet to be fully elucidated and may well differ depending on the nature of the reported memory alteration and the characteristics of the individual. Nevertheless, these findings have fueled much of the current public debate about recovered memories, so we turn now to a discussion of their limitations.

Some Limitations to the Misinformation Effect

To support their claims, critics of the veracity of recovered memories have relied heavily on the misinformation effects found by cognitive psychologists. But, we question the direct application of these experimental findings to clinical phenomena both because of the generalizability issues we raised earlier in this chapter (incomparable settings, measures, manipulations, and subjects) and because we believe that there are important limitations to these effects. Referring again to Mook (1983) and his suggestion that what laboratory research does best is illuminate "what can happen, rather than what typically does happen," the following section outlines some of the limitations of the misinformation effects and challenges some of the claims made about them.

In cognitive psychology, the focus is on understanding mental processes such as memory—processes common to all of us. The emphasis is on identifying and understanding the operation of fundamental mechanisms, for example, the conditions that enhance or undermine the encoding, storage, or retrieval of memories. Researchers are seeking universal effects (i.e., what is generally true across individuals). To the degree that they identify such general processes and basic mechanisms, they can make general claims.

This experimental focus on basic processes and mechanisms is typified in the following—not completely facetious—statement of Loftus and Hoffman (1989):

> We believe that the misinformation effect is sufficiently pervasive and eventually may be so highly controllable that we are tempted to propose a Watsonian future for the misinformation effect (see Watson 1939, p. 104, cited in Loftus and Hoffman 1989): Give us a dozen healthy memories, well-formed, and our own specified world to handle them in. And we'll guarantee to take any one at random and train it to become any type of memory that we might select—hammer, screwdriver, wrench, stop sign, yield sign, Indian chief—regardless of its origin or the brain that holds it. (p. 103)

In other words, the authors have found their evidence compelling enough to make an expansive claim and prediction about its generalizability.

More recently, the misinformation findings (now including the memory implantation results) have led Garry and Loftus (1994) to conclude that "it is not hard at all to make people truly believe they have seen or experienced something they have not" (pp. 365–366). This broad claim, we believe, lays the foundation for many of the attacks on memory recovery. However, does it really summarize or do justice to the empirical evidence? Let us examine it. (We undertake this exercise not for the sake of quarrelsomeness, but because this particular statement summarizes so many of the issues that we believe deserve further discussion.)

"It is not hard at all . . . "   How difficult is it? First, note that the misinformation findings are consistently rather small, implicating only a minority of subjects (0%–34%; typically fewer than one-quarter of adult subjects tested show them). (In all fairness, this clause may instead have been intended to convey the reliability of the findings rather than their generalizability—although we doubt this, given the previous "Watsonian" claim.) In contrast, consider an analogy in the clinical domain. It is unlikely that researchers would claim that "it is not hard at all" to treat disorder X, if only one-quarter of patients responded to the treatment. This contrast in what is considered an appropriate claim is, we believe, grounded in a fundamental difference in the two research traditions.

The experimental focus on identifying basic processes or mechanisms embraces statistical significance as the measure of the meaningfulness of a finding, sometimes irrespective of its real-world implications. In clinical research, *statistically significant* and *clinically significant* are distinct terms—the latter is a more stringent and appropriate criterion for clinical issues. In other words, as William James observed, the difference has to make a difference to be a difference. For example, in treatment outcomes, a drug is judged not only by whether it ameliorates symptoms to a statistically significant degree but also by whether treated patients show a reliable change from dysfunction to functionality (i.e., ideally, after treatment, patients should fall within the normal range; e.g., Ogles et al. 1995). These two contrasting research agendas serve their respective goals and need not conflict. They will conflict, however, if their limits are not specified. For the reasons described above, extreme caution must be used in generalizing from limited findings derived under such artificial circumstances to discussions of false memory creation in therapy.

" . . . to make people . . . "   Who is susceptible? Obviously, based on the preceding, we believe it would be more prudent to say "to make *some* people"; however, another issue is involved. The experimental focus on identifying basic processes or mechanisms also tends to ignore the possible role of specific characteristics of the individual in mediating the effect (i.e., "which people?"). The question of which people are vulnerable to misinformation effects seems a reasonable one to pose, given that only a limited proportion of subjects succumb to the effect. In other words, why them and why only them?

Experimentalists might argue that the numbers merely reflect the limits of their present knowledge and technique in instilling misleading information (as the "Watsonian" quote above would suggest) or the limitations inherent in single trial designs (G. Bower, personal communication, April 1996). However, alternative explanations are also possible. For example, if the misinformation effects actually represent reporting differences caused by factors such as compliance, suggestibility (D. Spiegel 1995), demand characteristics, or "misinformation acceptance" (subjects trusting the experimenters' information over their own memories) rather than actual memory alterations (for discussions, see Ceci and Bruck 1993; Loftus and Hoffman 1989; Zaragoza and Koshmider 1989), then individual differences in traits related to these factors could illuminate who would be susceptible to the effect—that is, what is it about those subjects?

Two recent findings lend credence to the reasonableness of this query and indicate that some experimentalists have begun to ask such questions. In a replication of Hyman et al.'s (1995) study, Hyman and Billings (unpublished, reported in Loftus et al., in press) found that hypnotizability/vividness of mental imagery and the tendency to have dissociative experiences were strongly correlated with the experimental implantation of false childhood memories. As we mentioned earlier in this chapter, hypnotizability is a known risk factor for the creation of pseudomemories (for discussions, see D. Brown 1995; D. Spiegel 1995). Consider also the Pezdek (1995) finding in which the implantation of false memories seemed to depend on the subject's degree of experience or knowledge about the nature of the event being implanted. In the case of a rectal enema, for which most subjects had a limited prior knowledge base, none of the attempted implantations was successful. The findings of Hyman and Billings and of Pezdek suggest that trait or knowledge differences may well play a role in the development of false memories. By asking and answering the question "What is it about those subjects?" with experimental and clinical research, we may begin to be able to predict with greater precision who is at risk for implantation of false memories. This development would bring a level of specificity to this literature that has been sorely lacking.

"... truly believe ... "   How truly are false beliefs held? There is little question that this issue is still the crux of significant debate. In a replication of the classic misinformation paradigm (Loftus et al. 1978), Zaragoza and Koshmider (1989) examined whether subjects exposed to misleading postevent information actually come to believe that they remember seeing that information at the time of the original event (i.e., that the memory is actually altered). They found that misled subjects were no more likely than subjects who were not misled to actually believe that they remembered seeing the misinformation as part of the original event. In addition, postevent exposure to misleading information did not reduce subjects' ability to accurately identify the original source of the information (i.e., they were no more likely to make source confusion errors). Zaragoza and Koshmider concluded that reporting misinformation does not necessarily indicate that subjects remember seeing it or have come to believe it to be true, and they note several possible alternative explanations for the misinformation effect (see also Loftus and Hoffman 1989). When a subject *does not* remember the original detail (e.g., that it was a stop sign), he or she may come to believe that the yield sign, introduced in the postevent information, was part of the original event either because it was introduced by a source that presumably has accurate information (the experimenter) or because the information simply fills a gap (and therefore does not conflict with anything) in his or her memory. Subjects who *do* remember the original detail may also report the misinformation either because it was offered by the experimenter, and they trust that source more than their own memory (*misinformation acceptance;* Loftus and Hoffman 1989), or because of social desirability or experimental demand characteristics (e.g., being cooperative, perceptions of how to do well on the test).

Likewise, in the study of implanting memories of fictional events in children, Ceci and his colleagues (1994) concede that it is impossible to determine from their data the degree to which any or all of the following factors contributed to the children's false reports: repeatedly being asked to think about the fictional event, being told that one's mother said that the event occurred, or repeatedly being asked to create images of the event. (In a footnote, they report that few children assent to fictional events if they are not given either of the latter two instructions.) The authors stated that "notwithstanding this inability to provide explanation, we do believe that not all false assenting reflected children's actual beliefs in the false events, because some children recanted these false assents after being told they were wrong in the final session" (Ceci et al. 1994, p. 317). In other words, the misinformation findings may well represent influences other than the alteration of true beliefs.

" . . . they have seen or experienced something they have not." How false is the false belief? Again, we refer to the studies previously described and note that the Pezdek study (1995) offers preliminary but suggestive evidence that a specific knowledge base may indeed be necessary before subjects can be convinced that have experienced something they have not (i.e., they must have some kind of experience of it already).

In the interests of clarity and circumspection then, we suggest that the statement, "It is not hard at all to make people truly believe they have seen or experienced something they have not," might be better rephrased as "It is possible to make some people mistakenly report that they have seen or experienced some things under certain (experimental) circumstances."

A Reconsideration of the Misinformation Effect

What do the misinformation and suggestibility effects reported by Loftus, Bruck, Ceci, and their colleagues in the experimental studies described above suggest? If we agree, as we do, that some memories could be altered or inserted in some people, what does it really tell us with respect to our considerations of recovered memory? For one thing, these findings underscore the necessity for significant caution in using suggestive "memory recovery" techniques in therapeutic situations, particularly with patients who have no memory of the abuse (for an extensive review, see Lindsay and Read 1994). These findings also offer some possible ways in which false or distorted memories "recovered" in therapy may be created (although, as we have emphasized, what a "false memory" actually represents—be it actual memory alteration, demand characteristics affecting reporting, or a belief in the new information rather than an actual memory of the implanted event—is far from established).

However, do these findings really challenge the credibility of recovered memories per se? Are they applicable to individuals who recover memories of childhood sexual abuse outside of a "recovered memory" therapy context? The factors that argue for the generalizability of experimental findings to therapy offices (such as suggestion of past events, perceived authority of the source, repetition of suggestions, perceived plausibility of suggestions, mental rehearsal, guided imagery, use of hypnosis; Lindsay and Read 1994) are less apparent in other settings where therapy is not involved (e.g., Stanton 1995), and therefore the generalizability argument seems uncomfortably stretched in these instances. Some experimentalists acknowledge this; for example, Lindsay and Read (1994) caution, in the beginning of their review, that their comments "are directed only to recollections of abuse that are the products of extensive use of memory recovery techniques and ancillary practices. People who have always remembered being sexually abused as children, or who spontaneously come to remember previously forgotten abuse, are on those bases different from clients who require months of guidance and memory recovery techniques prior to their first recollection" (p. 282). The possibility that some recovered memories may be created does not imply that all recovered memories are, in fact, created. Indeed, the experimental findings seem to be a rather clear example of experimental research showing what can happen rather than what typically does happen.

D. Spiegel (1995) offered an alternative conceptualization of what the misinformation studies may be revealing about memory. The fact that memory is malleable and subject to internal needs for comprehensibility and consistency and/or external suggestions and pressures is in no way inconsistent with the notion that traumatic memories may be dissociated or repressed. Contrary to the common assumption that these memory alteration findings are sufficient grounds for attacking the veracity of recovered memories, these studies may provide additional converging evidence in support of the possibility of dissociated memories, such as those seen in traumatic amnesia.

As a matter of pure logic, it should be equally easy to insert false information or to suppress true information (D. Spiegel 1995). Indeed, the former often requires the latter. The misinformation effect studies (reviewed in Garry and Loftus 1994) and the suggestion study of Bruck and associates (1995) offer cases in point. It may be argued that "to falsely remember a stop sign in an automobile accident, it is necessary to suppress veridical recollection of the yield sign that was there" (D. Spiegel 1995, p. 139). Similarly, for the misled children in the Bruck study to report remembering less crying at the time of the inoculation or to misidentify who gave them their shot suggests that the misinformation may be supplanting what they really remembered. This argument, however, requires that a true memory did exist and would have been reported if the postevent suggestions had not been inserted. Otherwise, it could be argued that the new information suggested by the questioner simply filled a memory gap, as in the Laurence and Perry (1983) "noises in the night" study (see also McCloskey and Zaragoza 1985), and would not be evidence of prior memories being displaced.

On this point, Loftus et al. (1978, p. 27) reported that, for at least half of their subjects, the initial information "got into memory in the first place" (i.e., they encoded the street sign). In the Bruck et al. (1995) study of children's memories for inoculations, reports of the amount of crying at 1 week and 1 year were highly stable for those children who were not given pain-denying feedback, and children who had not been misled about the actions of the pediatrician or research assistant were highly accurate about events for which they had memories. In other words, their memories for the event were intact—and could have been reported had they not been influenced—which suggests that those memories were suppressed at some level so that the suggested misinformation could be reported instead. This latter experiment is a particularly cogent example of the fact that misinformation is a two-edged sword: it may suppress veridical memories of traumatic experiences or create pseudomemories of traumatic experiences under certain circumstances. Additionally, the dissociation argument requires not only that a memory be supplanted but also that it remain retrievable. Zaragoza and Koshmider's (1989) finding, that subjects fed misleading information are not impaired in their ability to identify the original information, is consistent with this (i.e., the memory remains somewhere).

Conclusion

We discussed two large empirical literatures describing the effects of negative emotion and misinformation on memory. The issues we have examined urge use of caution in making inferences from experimental research to the clinical situation. Laboratory studies and surveys with nonclinical subjects indicate that negative affect tends to enhance memory, particularly for central details of an event. We considered several issues concerning the applicability of these research findings to clinical populations. In particular, we described some ways in which laboratory manipulations of emotion and memory appear to lack the "necessary nearness to life" (Stern 1910, p. 270, quoted in Yuille and Cutshall 1986, p. 291) that would allow the findings to be extrapolated to clinical populations with significant traumatic memories. This is important because the experimental findings seem to be at odds with the well-established clinical literature describing significant disturbances in memory associated with trauma. We also described several normal memory failure explanations that have been offered to account for traumatic amnesia and memory recovery—clinical phenomena that are often attributed to psychopathological processes of dissociation or repression. In this discussion, we concluded that these explanations are contradicted by the predictions that might be reasonably made about the memorability of events such as childhood sexual abuse. Furthermore, these explanations appear inadequate when measured up to the significance and extensiveness of the traumatic amnesia that they seek to explain.

The misinformation literature suggests that some memories (or reports of them) may be altered by postevent information or may even be implanted anew, both with and without hypnosis. We noted that the implications of misinformation effects for recovered memories are far from clear. These misinformation effects, real and important ones, may apply to only a minority of the population that has to date been little characterized—although recent studies indicate that suggestibility and proneness to dissociation may be predisposing factors. The literature also suggests that distortion of memory is most likely to occur when schemata similar to the imposed information preexist. Thus, those who are most likely to create false memories of trauma are those who also have real memories of it or elaborate (perhaps vicariously learned) schemata for it. The actual mechanisms and, therefore, meaning of the effects—whether the memory or the report is altered—have also not been established. To the extent that current social influence over memory retrieval distorts memory, such effects may occur in nature, as when an abusing parent denies to the child that the abuse occurred or threatens the child if she or he talks about it. Moreover, because both cognitive and social influences may be considerable in the therapist's office, clinicians should note the general cautions implied by these findings. We proposed that the misinformation phenomenon may be seen as consistent with the mechanisms of dissociation or repression, in that it requires the supplanting of one memory with another, particularly in cases in which the original information may still be reported. Misinformation pressure may as easily suppress as create traumatic memory. Misinformation may, then, be the other side of the coin of dissociation and repression.

Loftus and colleagues stated that "cognitive psychologists who question the idea of repressed and recovered memories naturally want some empirical evidence" (Garry et al. 1994, p. 449). We agree with the sentiment; however, given the ethical limitations on experimentally manipulating dissociation, memory implantation, or memory recovery of truly traumatic events, we need to find the reasonable balance between what laboratory analog studies offer as explanations of what may be happening and what clinical research and observation offer as descriptions of what is happening. In addition, the development of programmatic research dedicated to investigating these topics by, for example, using closer approximations of the clinical phenomena in the laboratory and by investigating some of the classic experimental findings with clinical subjects could yield findings that span the present information gap between these two disciplines.

References

American Psychiatric Association: Diagnostic and Statistical Manual of Mental Disorders, 3rd Edition, Revised. Washington, DC, American Psychiatric Association, 1987

American Psychiatric Association: Diagnostic and Statistical Manual of Mental Disorders, 4th Edition. Washington, DC, American Psychiatric Association, 1994

Bannister D: Psychology as an exercise in paradox. Bulletin of the British Psychological Society 19:21–26, 1966

Bartlett FC: Remembering: A Study in Experimental and Social Psychology. Cambridge, MA, Cambridge University Press, 1932

Beitchman JH, Zucker KJ, DaCosta GA, et al: A review of the long-term effects of child sexual abuse. Child Abuse Negl 16:101–118, 1992

Bower GH: Awareness, the unconscious, and repression: an experimental psychologist's perspective, in Repression and Dissociation—Implications for Personality Theory, Psychopathology, and Health. Edited by Singer JL. Chicago, IL, The University of Chicago Press, 1990, pp 209–231

Bower GH: Mood congruity of social judgments, in Emotion and Social Judgments. Edited by Forgas JP. Oxford, UK, Pergamon, 1991, pp 31–53

Bowman ES: Delayed memories of child abuse, part I: an overview of research findings on forgetting, remembering, and corroborating trauma. Dissociation (in press a)

Bowman ES: Delayed memories of child abuse, part II: an overview of research findings relevant to understanding their reliability and suggestibility. Dissociation (in press b)

Bremner JD, Scott TM, Delaney RC, et al: Deficits in short-term memory in posttraumatic stress disorder. Am J Psychiatry 150:1015–1019, 1993

Bremner JD, Bennett A, Southwick AM, et al: Toward a cognitive neuroscience of dissociation and altered memory functions in post-traumatic stress disorder, in Neurobiological and Clinical Consequences of Stress: From Normal Adaptation to Post
Traumatic Stress Disorder. Edited by Freidman MJ, Charney DS, Deutch AY. Philadelphia, PA, JB Lippincott, 1995a, pp 239–271

Bremner JD, Randall P, Scott TM, et al: MRI-based measurement of hippocampal volume
in patients with combat-related posttraumatic stress disorder. Am J Psychiatry
152:973–981, 1995b

Brett EA, Ostroff R: Imagery and posttraumatic stress disorder: an overview. Am J Psychiatry 142:417–424, 1985

Briere J, Conte J: Self-reported amnesia for abuse in adults molested as children. J Trauma
Stress 6:21–31, 1993

Brockway S: Case report: flashback as a post-traumatic stress disorder (PTSD) symptom
in a World War II veteran. Mil Med 153:372–373, 1988

Brown D: Pseudomemories: the standard of science and the standard of care in trauma
treatment. Am J Clin Hypn 37:1–24, 1995

Brown R, Kulik J: Flashbulb memories. Cognition 5:73–99, 1977

Bruck M, Ceci SJ, Francoeur E, et al: "I hardly cried when I got my shot!" Influencing
children's reports about a visit to their pediatrician. Child Dev 66:193–208, 1995

Burke A, Heuer F, Reisberg D: Remembering emotional events. Memory and Cognition
20:277–290, 1992

Butler LD, Duran REF, Jasiukaitis P, et al: Hypnotizability and traumatic experience: a
diathesis-stress model of dissociative symptomatology. Am J Psychiatry 153
(suppl):42–63, 1996

Ceci SJ, Bruck M: Suggestibility of the child witness: a historical review and synthesis.
Psychol Bull 113:403–439, 1993

Ceci SJ, Loftus EL, Leichtman MD, et al: The possible role of source misattributions in the
creation of false beliefs among preschoolers. Int J Clin Exp Hypn 42:304–320, 1994

Christianson S-A: Emotional stress and eyewitness memory: a critical review. Psychol Bull
112:284–309, 1992

Christianson S, Hubinette B: Hands up! A study of witnesses' emotional reactions and
memories associated with bank robberies. Applied Cognitive Psychology 7:365–379, 1993

Christianson S-A, Loftus EF: Memory for traumatic events. Applied Cognitive Psychology
1:225–239, 1987

Christianson S-A, Loftus EF: Some characteristics of people's traumatic memories. Bulletin of the Psychonomic Society 28:195–198, 1990

Easterbrook JA: The effect of emotion on cue utilization and the organization of behavior.
Psychol Rev 66:183–201, 1959

Ellenberger HF: The Discovery of the Unconscious: The History and Evolution of Dynamic Psychiatry. New York, Basic Books, 1970

Elliot DM, Briere J: Posttraumatic stress associated with delayed recall of sexual abuse: a
general population study. J Trauma Stress 8:629–647, 1995

Elliot DM, Fox B: Child abuse and amnesia: prevalence and triggers to memory recovery.
Poster presented at the annual meeting of the International Society of Traumatic Stress
Studies, Chicago, IL, November 1994, pp 1–8

Feldman-Summers S, Pope KS: The experience of "forgetting" childhood abuse: a national
survey of psychologists. J Consult Clin Psychol 62:636–639, 1994

Finkelhor D: The trauma of child sexual abuse: two models. Journal of Interpersonal Violence 2:348–366, 1988

Finkelhor D, Hotaling G, Lewis IA, et al: Sexual abuse in a national survey of adult men
and women: prevalence, characteristics, and risk factors. Child Abuse Negl 14:19–28,
1990

Freud S: Remembering, repeating and working-through (further recommendations on
the technique of psycho-analysis II) (1914), in The Standard Edition of the Complete
Psychological Works of Sigmund Freud, Vol 12. Translated and edited by Strachey J.
London, Hogarth Press, 1958, pp 145–156

Freyd JJ: Theoretical and personal perspectives on the delayed memory debate. Paper presented at The Center for Mental Health at Foote Hospital's Continuing Education Conference: Controversies Around Recovered Memories of Incest and Ritualistic Abuse, Ann Arbor, MI, August 1993, pp 1–40

Ganaway GK: Historical versus narrative truth: clarifying the role of exogenous trauma in the etiology of MPD and its variants. Dissociation 2:205–220, 1989

Garry M, Loftus EF: Pseudomemories without hypnosis. Int J Clin Exp Hypn 42:363–378, 1994

Garry M, Loftus EF, Brown SW: Memory: a river runs through it. Consciousness and Cognition 3:438–451, 1994

Goldfield AE, Mollica RF, Pesavento BH, et al: The physical and psychological sequelae of torture: symptomatology and diagnosis. JAMA 259:2725–2729, 1988

Green BL: Psychosocial research in traumatic stress: an update. J Trauma Stress 7:341–362, 1994

Grinker RR, Spiegel JP: Men Under Stress. Philadelphia, PA, Blakiston, 1945

Harvey MR, Herman JL: Amnesia, partial amnesia, and delayed recall among adult survivors of childhood trauma. Consciousness and Cognition 3:295–306, 1994

Herman JL, Schatzow E: Recovery and verification of memories of childhood sexual trauma. Psychoanalytic Psychology 4:1–14, 1987

Hilgard ER: Hypnotic Susceptibility. New York, Harcourt Brace Jovanovich, 1965

Horowitz MJ: Stress Response Syndromes. New York, Jason Aronson, 1986

Hyman IE, Husband TH, Billings FJ: False memories of childhood experiences. Applied Cognitive Psychology 9:181–197, 1995

Ingram RE: External validity issues in mood and memory research. Journal of Social Behavior and Personality 4:57–62, 1989

Jaffe R: Dissociative phenomena in former concentration camp inmates. Int J Psychoanal 49:310–312, 1968

Janet P: The Major Symptoms of Hysteria. London, MacMillan, 1907

Kardiner A: The Traumatic Neuroses of War. New York, Basic Books, 1941

Kardiner A, Spiegel H: War Stress and Neurotic Illness. New York, Paul Hoeber, 1947

Kassin SM, Ellsworth PC, Smith VL: The "general acceptance" of psychological research on eyewitness testimony: a survey of the experts. Am Psychol 44:1089–1098, 1989

Kihlstrom JF: Hypnosis, delayed recall, and the principles of memory. Int J Clin Exp Hypn 42:337–345, 1994

Koopman C, Classen C, Spiegel D: Predictors of posttraumatic stress symptoms among survivors of the Oakland/Berkeley, Calif., firestorm. Am J Psychiatry 151:888–894, 1994

Krystal JH, Bremner JD, Southwick SM, et al: The emerging neurobiology of dissociation: implications for the treatment of PTSD, in Trauma, Memory and Dissociation. Edited by Bremner JD, Marmar C. Washington, DC, American Psychiatric Press (in press)

Kuehn LL: Looking down a gun barrel: person perception and violent crime. Percept Mot Skills 39:1159–1164, 1974

Laurence JR, Perry C: Hypnotically created memory among highly hypnotizable subjects. Science 222:523–524, 1983

Laurence JR, Nadon R, Nogrady H, et al: Duality, dissociation, and memory creation in highly hypnotizable subjects. Int J Clin Exp Hypn 34:295–310, 1986

Lindsay DS, Read JD: Psychotherapy and memories of childhood sexual abuse: a cognitive perspective. Applied Cognitive Psychology 8:281–338, 1994

Loftus EF: Leading questions and the eyewitness report. Cognitive Psychology 7:560–572, 1975

Loftus EF: The reality of repressed memories. Am Psychol 48:518–537, 1993

Loftus EF, Burns T: Mental shock can produce retrograde amnesia. Memory and Cognition 10:318–323, 1982

Loftus EF, Hoffman HG: Misinformation and memory: the creation of new memories. J Exp Psychol Gen 118:100–104, 1989

Loftus EF, Ketcham K: The Myth of Repressed Memories. New York, St Martin's Press, 1994

Loftus EF, Palmer JC: Reconstruction of automobile destruction: an example of the interaction between language and memory. Journal of Verbal Learning and Verbal Behavior 13:585–589, 1974

Loftus EF, Pickrell JE: The formation of false memories. Psychiatric Annals 25:720–725, 1995

Loftus EF, Miller DG, Burns HJ: Semantic integration of verbal information into a visual memory. J Exp Psychol Hum Learn 4:19–31, 1978

Loftus EF, Loftus GR, Messo J: Some facts about "weapon focus." Law and Human Behavior 11:55–62, 1987

Loftus EF, Garry M, Feldman J: Forgetting sexual trauma: what does it mean when 38% forget? J Consult Clin Psychol 62:1177–1181, 1994a

Loftus EF, Polonsky S, Fullilove MT: Memories of childhood sexual abuse: remembering and repressing. Psychology of Women Quarterly 18:67–84, 1994b

Loftus EF, Coan JA, Pickrell JE: Manufacturing false memories using bits of reality, in Implicit Memory and Metacognition. Edited by Reder L. Hillsdale, NJ, Lawrence Erlbaum (in press)

Lynn SJ, Rhue JW, Myers BP, et al: Pseudomemory in hypnotized and simulating subjects. Int J Clin Exp Hypn 42:118–129, 1994

Maldonado JR, Spiegel D: The treatment of post-traumatic stress disorder, in Dissociation: Clinical and Theoretical Perspectives. Edited by Lynn SJ, Rhue JW. New York, Guilford, 1994, pp 215–241

Marmar CR, Weiss DS, Schlenger WE, et al: Peritraumatic dissociation and posttraumatic stress in male Vietnam theater veterans. Am J Psychiatry 151:902–907, 1994

McCloskey M, Zaragoza M: Misleading postevent information and memory for events: arguments and evidence against memory impairment hypotheses. J Exp Psychol Gen 114:1–16, 1985

McCloskey M, Wible CG, Cohen NJ: Is there a special flashbulb-memory mechanism? J Exp Psychol Gen 117:171–181, 1988

Mook DG: In defense of external validity. Am Psychol 38:379–387, 1983

Morgan AH, Hilgard ER: Age differences in susceptibility to hypnosis. Int J Clin Exp Hypn 21:78–85, 1973

Mueser KT, Butler RW: Auditory hallucinations in combat-related chronic posttraumatic stress disorder. Am J Psychiatry 144:299–302, 1987

Murdock BB: Human Memory: Theory and Data. Potomac, MD, Lawrence Erlbaum, 1974

Neisser U: Snapshots or benchmarks?, in Memory Observed. Edited by Neisser U. San Francisco, CA, WH Freeman, 1982, pp 43–48

Nelson K: The psychological and social origins of autobiographical memory. Psychological Science 4:7–14, 1993

Ofshe RJ, Singer MT: Recovered-memory therapy and robust repression: influence and pseudomemories. Int J Clin Exp Hypn 42:391–410, 1994

Ofshe RJ, Watters E: Making Monsters: False Memory, Psychotherapy, and Sexual Hysteria. New York, Scribners, 1994

Ogles BM, Lambert MJ, Sawyer JD: Clinical significance of the National Institute of Mental Health Treatment of Depression Collaborative Research Program data. J Consult Clin Psychol 63:321–326, 1995

Olio KA, Cornell WF: Making meaning not monsters: reflections on the delayed memory controversy. Journal of Child Sexual Abuse 3:77–94, 1994

Pezdek K: What types of false childhood memories are not likely to be suggestively implanted? Paper presented at the meeting of the Psychonomic Society, Los Angeles, CA, November 1–23, 1995

Piaget J: Paleys, Dreams and Imitation in Childhood. New York, WW Norton, 1962

Piccione C, Hilgard ER, Zimbardo PG: On the degree of stability of measured hypnotizability over a 25-year period. J Pers Soc Psychol 56:289–295, 1989

Pillemer DB: Flashbulb memories of the assassination attempt on President Reagan. Cognition 16:63–84, 1984

Polusny MA, Follette VM: Long term correlates of child sexual abuse: theory and review of the empirical literature. Applied and Preventative Psychology 4:143–166, 1995

Polusny MA, Follette VM: Remembering childhood sexual abuse: a national survey of psychologists' clinical practices, beliefs, and personal experiences. Professional Psychology: Research and Practice 27:41–52, 1996

Pope HG, Hudson JI: Does childhood sexual abuse cause adult psychiatric disorder? Essentials of methodology. Journal of Psychiatry and Law 23:363–381, 1995

Pynoos RS, Nader K: Children's memory and proximity of violence. J Am Acad Child Adolesc Psychiatry 28:236–241, 1989

Pynoos RS, Frederick C, Nader K, et al: Life threat and posttraumatic stress in school-age children. Arch Gen Psychiatry 44:1057–1063, 1987

Rowan AB, Foy DW: Post-traumatic stress disorder in child sexual abuse survivors: a literature review. J Trauma Stress 6:3–19, 1993

Rowan AB, Foy DW, Rodriguez N, et al: Posttraumatic stress disorder in a clinical sample of adults sexually abused as children. Child Abuse Negl 18:51–61, 1994

Russell DEH: The incidence and prevalence of intrafamilial and extrafamilial sexual abuse of female children. Child Abuse Negl 7:133–146, 1983

Schacter DL: Implicit memory: history and current status. J Exp Psychol Learn Mem Cogn 13:510–518, 1987

Schacter D: Understanding implicit memory: a cognitive neuroscience approach. Am Psychol 47:559–569, 1992

Schacter D, Moscovitch M: Infants, amnesia, and dissociable memory systems, in Infant Memory. Edited by Moscovitch M. New York, Plenum, 1984, pp 173–216

Siegel DJ: Memory, trauma, and psychotherapy. Journal of Psychotherapy Practice and Research 4:93–122, 1995

Spanos NP, Menary E, Gabora NJ, et al: Secondary identity enactments during hypnotic past-life regression: a sociocognitive perspective. J Pers Soc Psychol 61:308–320, 1991

Spanos NP, Burgess CA, Burgess MF: Past-life identities, UFO abductions, and satanic ritual abuse: the social construction of memories. Int J Clin Exp Hypn 42:433–446, 1994

Spiegel D: Multiple personality as a post-traumatic stress disorder. Psychiatr Clin North Am 7:101–110, 1984

Spiegel D: Dissociating damage. Am J Clin Hypn 29:123–131, 1986

Spiegel D: The use of hypnosis in the treatment of PTSD. Psychiatr Med 10:21–30, 1992

Spiegel D: Hypnosis and suggestion, in Memory Distortion—How Minds, Brains, and Societies Reconstruct the Past. Edited by Schacter DL. Cambridge, MA, Harvard University Press, 1995, pp 129–149

Spiegel D, Cardeña E: Dissociative mechanisms in posttraumatic stress disorder, in Posttraumatic Stress Disorder: Etiology, Phenomenology, and Treatment. Edited by Wolf ME, Mosnaim AD. Washington, DC, American Psychiatric Press, 1990, pp 22–34

Spiegel D, Cardeña E: Disintegrated experience: the dissociative disorders revisited. J Abnorm Psychol 100:366–378, 1991

Spiegel H, Spiegel D: Trance and Treatment: Clinical Uses of Hypnosis. Washington, DC, American Psychiatric Press, 1987

Squire LR: Memory and the hippocampus: a synthesis from findings with rats, monkeys, and humans. Psychol Rev 99:195–231, 1992

Stanton M: Bearing witness: a man's recovery of his sexual abuse as a child. Providence Journal-Bulletin, May 7–9, 1995, pp 1A and following

Tellegen A: Practicing the two disciplines for relaxation and enlightenment: comment on "Role of the feedback signal in electromyograph biofeedback: the relevance of attention" by Qualls and Sheehan. J Exp Psychol Gen 110:217–226, 1981

Tellegen A, Atkinson G: Openness to absorbing and self-altering experiences ("absorption"), a trait related to hypnotic susceptibility. J Abnorm Psychol 83:268–277, 1974

Terr L: What happens to early memories of trauma? A study of twenty children under age five at the time of documented traumatic events. J Am Acad Child Adolesc Psychiatry 27:96–104, 1988

Terr L: Childhood traumas: an outline and overview. Am J Psychiatry 148:10–20, 1991

Tromp S, Koss MP, Figueredo AJ, et al: Are rape memories different? A comparison of rape, other unpleasant, and pleasant memories among employed women. J Trauma Stress 8:607–627, 1995

Tulving E, Thompson DM: Encoding specificity and retrieval processes in episodic memory. Psychol Rev 80:352–373, 1973

van der Hart O, Spiegel D: Hypnotic assessment and treatment of trauma-induced psychoses: the early psychotherapy of H. Breukink and modern views. Int J Clin Exp Hypn 41:191–209, 1993

van der Kolk BA: Psychological Trauma. Washington, DC, American Psychiatric Press, 1987

van der Kolk BA, Ducey CR: The psychological processing of traumatic experience: Rorschach patterns in PTSD. J Trauma Stress 2:259–274, 1989

van der Kolk BA, Fisler R: Dissociation and the fragmentary nature of traumatic memories: overview and exploratory study. J Trauma Stress 8:505–525, 1995

van der Kolk BA, Kadish W: Amnesia, dissociation, and the return of the repressed, in Psychological Trauma. Edited by van der Kolk BA. Washington, DC, American Psychiatric Press, 1987, pp 173–190

van der Kolk BA, van der Hart O: Pierre Janet and the breakdown of adaptation in psychological trauma. Am J Psychiatry 146:1530–1540, 1989

van der Kolk BA, van der Hart O: The intrusive past: the flexibility of memory and the engraving of trauma. American Imago 48:425–454, 1991

van der Kolk BA, Blitz R, Burr W, et al: Nightmares and trauma: a comparison of nightmares after combat with lifelong nightmares in veterans. Am J Psychiatry 141:187–190, 1984

Wessel I, Merckelbach H: Characteristics of traumatic memories in normal subjects. Behavioral and Cognitive Psychotherapy 22:315–324, 1994

Wilkinson CB: Aftermath of a disaster: the collapse of the Hyatt Regency Hotel skywalks. Am J Psychiatry 140:1134–1139, 1983

Williams LM: Recall of childhood trauma: a prospective study of women's memories of child sexual abuse. J Consult Clin Psychol 62:1167–1176, 1994a

Williams LM: What does it mean to forget child sexual abuse? A reply to Loftus, Garry, and Feldman (1994). J Consult Clin Psychol 62:1182–1186, 1994b

Williams LM: Recovered memories of abuse in women with documented child victimization histories. J Trauma Stress 8:649–673, 1995

Wyatt G: The sexual abuse of Afro-American and white American women in childhood. Child Abuse Negl 9:507–519, 1985

Yerkes RM, Dodson JD: The relation of strength of stimulus to rapidity of habit-formation. Journal of Comparative Neurology and Psychology 18:459–482, 1908

Yuille JC, Cutshall JL: A case study of eyewitness memory of a crime. J Appl Psychol 71:291–301, 1986

Zaragoza M, Koshmider JW III: Misled subjects may know more than their performance implies. J Exp Psychol Learn Mem Cogn 15:246–255, 1989

Chapter 7

Memory, Repression, and Abuse: Recovered Memory and Confident Reporting of the Personal Past

Kevin M. McConkey, Ph.D.

Memory provides us with an account of the past, helps us operate in the present, and helps us prepare for the future. Sometimes our memories are perfect; sometimes they are not. Sometimes we recover memories and remember things that we had forgotten; sometimes we create accounts of events that we had never experienced. Memory is a constructive and reconstructive process that serves us reasonably well in everyday life but sometimes misleads us and others. The biological, cognitive, and social influences that shape memory are intertwined in the debate about recovered memory and confident reporting of the personal past. The problems of memory, repression, and abuse are at the core of this debate, which in recent years has polarized the psychiatric and psychological communities, as well as patients and their family members. In the civil war that is being fought over this issue in homes, clinics, laboratories, and courts—and reported on and fueled by the media—the focus is the validity of recovered memories of childhood sexual abuse.

In this debate, the central issue is neither the occurrence of nor the possible harm done by childhood sexual abuse. There is no question that sexual abuse during childhood may be associated with major physical and mental health problems during adulthood (e.g., Kendall-Tackett et al. 1993; Levitt and Pinnell 1995; Nash et al. 1993; Roesler and McKenzie 1994; Romans et al. 1995; Schulte et al. 1995; Walker et al. 1995). Also, the central issue is not the reporting of always held, but previously unreported, memories of childhood sexual abuse. There is no question that some individuals do not report childhood sexual abuse even though they have memories of that abuse (e.g., Femina et al. 1990;

Preparation of this chapter was supported in part by a grant to the author from the Australian Research Council. The author is grateful to Amanda Barnier, Karen Bishop, Richard Bryant, Jacquelyn Cranney, Fiona Maccallum, and David Spiegel for comments and assistance during its preparation.

Freyd 1994; Kuyken and Brewin 1995; Loftus et al. 1994a). Rather, the central issue is the reporting of recovered memories of childhood sexual abuse by adults who had not previously indicated any memories of abuse. For some, this type of reporting involves the therapeutic recovery of repressed true memories. For others, this type of reporting involves the iatrogenic creation of false memories.

In recent years, a large and rapidly increasing number of publications on memory, repression, and suggestion have appeared in the context of this debate about recovered and false memory. These include professional and popular books (e.g., Bass and Davis 1994; Blume 1990; Dawes 1994; Fredrickson 1992; Goldstein 1992; Goldstein and Farmer 1993; Herman 1992; Kaminer 1993; Loftus and Ketcham 1994; Lynn and Rhue 1994; MacLean 1993; McConkey and Sheehan 1995; Ofshe and Watters 1994; Pendergrast 1994; Singer 1990; Spiegel 1994; Terr 1994; Wright 1994; Yapko 1994), special issues of journals (e.g., *American Journal of Clinical Hypnosis* 36(3), 1996; *Applied Cognitive Psychology* 8(4), 1994; *Consciousness and Cognition* 3(3–4), 1994; *International Journal of Clinical and Experimental Hypnosis* 42(4), 1994, and 43(2), 1995; *Journal of Traumatic Stress* 8(4), 1995; *The Counseling Psychologist* 23(2), 1995), and major journal articles (e.g., Bloom 1994; Bowers and Farvolden 1996; Freyd 1994; Loftus 1993; Lynn and Nash 1994; McConkey 1995; Pope and Hudson 1995). This publication trend will continue. It is hoped, however, that a shift will occur toward more reasoned and reasonable positions than some of those seen in the literature to date. That shift will require the motivation, time, and effort of all of us, and, in that sense, it will be similar to the processes of both therapy and science.

With an overall aim of contributing to that shift, this chapter has three objectives: 1) to provide an evaluative summary of core concepts and selected findings, 2) to comment on the relevance for clinical practice of current knowledge, and 3) to indicate the preferred directions for research to expand current knowledge. With those objectives in mind, in this chapter, I discuss 1) memory and repression, 2) traumatic memory and recovered memory, 3) recovered memory and well-being, and 4) guidelines for practice and directions for research. At the outset, it is important to recognize the difficulties that are involved in presenting a balanced position on the issues associated with recovered memories of childhood sexual abuse (e.g., Banks and Pezdek 1994; Enns et al. 1995; Green 1995; Grossman and Pressley 1994; Lindsay 1994, 1995; Lindsay and Read 1994). Across the literature, there is wide variation, for instance, in definitions of abuse, trauma, and repression. In addition, there is wide variation in what is considered acceptable evidence for the occurrence and validity of recovered memories of childhood sexual abuse. Given the imprecision and variation on these and other issues, we should not underestimate the difficulties involved in finding common ground, but we should continue to try.

Memory and Repression

Memory experts agree on many issues, including the fact that memory can be accurate, fallible, incomplete, malleable, and susceptible to external factors. Each of these points of agreement and the psychological principles that underscore them can be documented in a variety of ways (e.g., Bekerian and Goodrich 1995; Kihlstrom 1994; Kihlstrom and Barnhardt 1993; Neisser and Fivush 1994). By its nature, memory is a constructive process that is influenced by a wide range of cognitive and social events (e.g., Bartlett 1932; Cialdini 1993), including information that is provided during the encoding of the original event, during the storage of that memory, and during the retrieval of that memory (e.g., Garry et al. 1994; Johnson and Raye 1981; Johnson et al. 1993; Weingardt et al. 1995). Moreover, the use of techniques such as hypnosis to enhance retrieval can lead to major changes in individuals' reported recall and in their confidence in the accuracy of their memory (Krass et al. 1988; McConkey 1992, 1995; McConkey and Sheehan 1995). Put simply, individuals can believe strongly in the accuracy of their hypnotically enhanced memories, even though those memories are inaccurate (e.g., Barnier and McConkey 1992; Nogrady et al. 1985). In terms of the use of hypnosis to enhance memory, McConkey (1992) concluded that "it should be understood clearly that the experimental findings provide no guarantee that any benefits (e.g., increased accurate recall) will be obtained through its use, and that some costs (e.g., inaccurate recall, inappropriate confidence) may well be incurred through its use" (p. 426).

Although hypnosis causes problematic effects on memory, it is important to note that these effects have been recognized by and documented in research. The research that is desperately needed to determine the precise positive and negative effects on memory of other memory enhancement techniques, such as journal keeping and group discussion, has not been done. We should not assume that such techniques are problem-free in terms of their effects on memory, but we should acknowledge that we do not know what the problems are. In addition to the problems of particular techniques, particular types of patients may be especially vulnerable to memory confusions. For example, Bryant (1995) observed a relationship between fantasy proneness and reports of childhood sexual abuse; in particular, reports of abuse at a younger age were associated with a higher level of fantasy proneness. This finding, as well as others (e.g., Lynn and Rhue 1988), indicates that fantasy proneness may be a central process variable involved in the reconstruction of memories of childhood sexual abuse and underscores that patients who are prone to fantasy engagement may be especially vulnerable to factors that lead to the creation of memories.

Although substantial research has established that memories are malleable and should not be accepted as self-validating, this research is sometimes rejected as irrelevant to the debate about recovered memory because it has not involved memory for severely traumatic events (e.g., Herman 1992; Olio 1989; Terr 1994; van der Kolk 1994). This rejection, however, misses the point of the research. Recognizing that memory is malleable does not mean that recovered memories of childhood sexual abuse are necessarily false; rather, it means that they are not necessarily accurate. Moreover, there is no reason that memory for traumatic events should follow entirely different psychological principles from those followed by memory for nontraumatic events. Although a case for that possibility is made by some (e.g., Terr 1994; van der Kolk and Fisler 1995), evidence indicates that traumatic memories can be influenced by the same range of cognitive and social events that influence nontraumatic memories (e.g., Foa et al. 1995; Garry and Loftus 1994; Ofshe and Singer 1994). Recognition of this latter point is especially needed because it should make clinicians think more carefully about the techniques used in therapy and the inferences drawn from memories reported during therapy.

The focus by some on the distinctiveness of memory for traumatic events is linked to the central role of the concept of repression in the debate about recovered memories of childhood sexual abuse (e.g., Herman 1992; Olio 1989; Terr 1994). Repression, in a general sense, involves the motivated forgetting of information that is threatening to the self (e.g., Bowers and Farvolden 1996; Erdelyi 1993; Singer 1990). Note, however, that there are many variants in conceptualizing repression and related constructs such as dissociation and that variation is one of the problems of this debate (e.g., Lynn and Rhue 1994; Singer 1990; Spiegel 1994). Moreover, analyses of the original concept of repression in the writings of Freud have typically highlighted its internal inconsistencies and its limited value beyond a very general description of assumed processes (e.g., Bowers and Farvolden 1996; Brenneis 1994; Crews 1996; Ganaway 1994, 1995; Macmillan 1991). Overall, the relative impreciseness of the concept of repression, and the difficulty in testing it, has led some to argue that it is theoretically meaningless and without scientific support (e.g., Holmes 1974, 1990). In his review of relevant empirical research, Holmes (1990), for instance, concluded that "despite over sixty years of research . . . there is no controlled laboratory evidence supporting the concept of repression" (p. 96) and suggested, perhaps only a little facetiously, that those who choose to continue using the notion should precede it with a warning that "the concept of repression has not been validated with experimental research and its use may be hazardous to the accurate interpretation of clinical behavior" (p. 97).

The limitations of the concept of repression (and of dissociation) must be recognized, but it is impossible to ignore the substantial amount of clinical observation and personal anecdote that point to the ways in which individuals can set aside or avoid thoughts and memories that are unpleasant or threatening to them (e.g., Bower 1990; Davis 1990; Erdelyi 1993; Freyd 1994; Nemiah 1984; Weinberger 1990). Careful clinical observation plays a central role in conceptualizing many ideas in the domain of psychopathology, and systematic clinical observation of unreported, forgotten, and repressed memories of childhood sexual abuse is needed. Thoughts about and memories of important personal events can be set aside from normal awareness, and a concept such as repression or dissociation is needed to help understand that process. Accepting the value of such a concept, however, does not necessarily require an acceptance of the accuracy of reports of those thoughts and memories. As Bowers and Farvolden (1996) noted, "Endorsing the concept of repression does not commit theorists to the belief that recovered memories must be historically accurate in all particulars. A memory, by virtue of having been repressed, does not somehow escape the distortions and constructive features of memories in general" (p. 361).

Despite clinical anecdotes, the repression or dissociation of a memory of a traumatic childhood event may be relatively rare. Indeed, it seems that traumatic events are more likely to lead to recurrent and intrusive memories, in which biological, cognitive, and social processes may be involved (e.g., Bremner et al. 1995; Cotton 1994; Frankel 1994; LeDoux 1991; LeDoux et al. 1989; Nash 1994; Schachter et al. 1995; van der Kolk 1994; van der Kolk and Fisler 1995; van der Kolk and Saporta 1991). The fact that we sometimes remember events that we had forgotten does not mean that those events were traumatic, nor does it mean that those particular memories were repressed. Much of the nonreporting of such events may occur because of normal forgetting, embarrassment about reporting the events, the consequences of reporting the events, or other reasons that relate to factors other than repression (e.g., Freyd 1994; Loftus 1993). Currently, we cannot "distinguish between those [patients] who do not recall actual abuse and those who do not report on it, and among the former, between memory failures that reflect repression, dissociation, and other pathological processes, and those that are benign" (Kihlstrom 1995, p. 66). In other words, we should not assume that newly reported material indicates the lifting of repression that is linked to negative emotional experiences of childhood. As Nash (1994) concluded,

> when we are faced with patients who experience themselves as suddenly and agonizingly remembering a previously forgotten trauma . . . we should above all else recognize the enormous clinical importance of this material . . . [but recognize also that] memories do not literally return in pristine form, unsullied by contemporary factors like suggestion, transference, values, social context, and fantasies elaborated at the time of (and subsequent to) the event. (p. 357)

Traumatic Memory and Recovered Memory

The effects of trauma on memory apparently can range from individuals "being overwhelmed with unbidden memories of past events to [their] having no memory at all of the traumatic event or any aspect thereof" (Green 1995, p. 502). Recent research on traumatic memory has included an examination of the breakdown of cognitive functioning when trauma is occurring (e.g., Nachmani 1995), the neuroanatomical correlates of stress on memory (e.g., Bremner et al. 1995), the characteristics of traumatic memories (e.g., van der Kolk and Fisler 1995), the retention of personal experiences by children and the effects of repeated questions on their recall (e.g., Fivush and Schwarzmueller 1995; Ornstein 1995), the nature of memories of female sexual assault and the influence of therapy on those memories (e.g., Foa et al. 1995; Tromp et al. 1995), and the use of traumatic memories in the clinical setting when they are known to be accurate or inaccurate (e.g., Fowler 1994; Nash 1994). I illustrate recent research by summarizing selected studies and drawing out the relevance of the findings.

Howe et al. (1994) studied the nature and onset of early personal memories for traumatic events. In an analysis of children's recall of emergency room treatment, these authors concluded that children younger than 2 years retained very limited memories and that coherent memories did not develop until a sense of self was established after that age. Moreover, they reported that the pattern of recall for traumatic events was essentially similar to that for nontraumatic events; specifically, over time there was a loss of detail, but a retention of the gist, for both types of events. Goodman et al. (1994) interviewed young children after they had undergone a stressful procedure involving urethral catheterization. The strongest findings were related to the relevance of age differences. In particular, younger (3–4 years old) rather than older (7–10 years old) children recalled less about their experience, answered fewer questions, and made more errors in their answers. Also, factors such as the child's comprehension of the event, the mother's attention at the time, the communication between mother and child, and the child's emotional reaction at the time influenced the memory of this stressful event (Goodman et al. 1994).

Ceci et al. (1994a; see also Ceci et al. 1994b) reported that the difficulty in separating two or more sources of memory was a powerful mechanism underlying children's false beliefs about experiencing particular events; specifically, some children misattributed the source of their memory about a fictitious event. These authors interviewed children about real (parent-supplied) and fictitious (experimenter-contrived) events, and these interviews were conducted 7–10 times at intervals of 7–10 days for each child. The authors reported that all children were susceptible to source misattributions, but the younger children were particularly vulnerable when they were exposed to interview techniques that involved the creation of a mental image of the fictitious event. Such techniques increased the likelihood that younger children would believe that they had experienced those events, when, in fact, they had only imagined them in fantasy. This finding is consistent with other research on the way in which visual imagery about an event tends to lead to a belief in the existence of the event, independent of its actual occurrence (e.g., Dobson and Markham 1993; Markham and Hynes 1993).

To examine the effect of interviewing techniques, Fivush (1994) investigated how young children's recall of events may be changed through discussion with others. She interviewed children at ages 40, 46, 58, and 70 months about personal events and found that the children tended to incorporate relatively little of the information provided by the interview into their subsequent recall; however, they were generally inconsistent in the information that they recounted at the various interview times. Fivush (1994) acknowledged that her study raised more questions than it answered about the extent to which young children are susceptible to leading questions or the extent to which they retain accurate memories of personal events.

Hyman et al. (1995) conducted two experiments to investigate the creation of false memories of childhood experiences in response to misleading information and repeated interviews. Parents were asked to provide information about events that had occurred during the subjects' childhood, and subjects were interviewed about these events and about other events that were created and suggested by the experimenter. In the experiments, either 20% or 25% of the subjects created false memories; moreover, those individuals who had discussed background events relevant to the suggested false memories were more likely to subsequently incorporate those false memories into their own reporting. That is, a general discussion opened the way for the planting of a false memory in some, but not all, of the individuals.

In recognition of the potential influence on reported memory of interviewing techniques, Saywitz and Moan-Hardie (1994) tested a procedure to reduce children's distortion of their memories. In particular, they asked children to stop and think before answering questions and allowed them to indicate whether or not they remembered. The findings indicated that when this procedure was used, acquiescence was reduced and resistance was increased to misleading questions. Saywitz and Moan-Hardie (1994) noted the potential value of adopting such a procedure when dealing with the recall of childhood trauma by adults.

The necessity and potential value of developing and using appropriate interview procedures must be underscored. This is especially so because, although existing procedures have been greatly criticized (e.g., Lindsay and Read 1994; Schooler 1994), there is relatively little guidance on the interview techniques that should be used to minimize distortion in the reporting of memories of childhood sexual abuse (Pennebaker and Memon 1996; however, see Fisher and Geiselman 1992; McConkey and Sheehan 1995). It would be helpful to the debate about recovered memory as a whole to shift away from indicating what should not be done in therapy to indicating more forcefully and in more detail what should be done and why. In this respect, therapists should use techniques that help patients consider and progress in a direct way with their present problems and their hopes for the future and should limit the degree to which they create an imbalance in the lives of patients by inappropriately focusing on uncertain events of the past. Therapists and patients should collaborate on the deeds of the future rather than the assumed misdeeds of the past. Moreover, therapists should convey clearly to patients that they can work effectively with them without becoming involved in debates about the personal past. Hearing and working with what patients say about their beliefs is quite different from encouraging and seeking to validate the patients' reported memories.

In terms of the characteristics of the traumatic memories reported by adults, van der Kolk and Fisler (1995) used a structured interview to question adults about a traumatic and a nontraumatic memory. They found that people reported experiences of traumatic memories in different ways from how they reported experiences of nontraumatic memories. In particular, these investigators observed that sensory modalities were more likely to be associated with the reporting of traumatic memories. Given this finding, they argued that traumatic memories are invariable and do not change over time because of the nature of the sensory information associated with them; however, they also considered that "once . . . the sensations are transcribed into a personal narrative they presumably become subject to the laws that govern explicit memory: to become a socially communicable story that is subject to condensation, embellishment, and contamination" (van der Kolk and Fisler 1995, p. 521).

In other work on the characteristics of traumatic memories, Tromp et al. (1995) surveyed women's memories of rape, other unpleasant events, and pleasant events. They found that unpleasant and pleasant memories differed in terms of a range of feelings and consequences and that rape memories differed from other unpleasant memories by being less clear and vivid, less well remembered, and less thought and talked about and by having a less meaningful order. This study raised important questions about the reasons that rape memories had these characteristics and also raised issues about the way in which memories of different types of events should be dealt with clinically.

In this respect, Foa et al. (1995) examined female rape victims in terms of the changes in their narratives of rape during therapy. They found that the length of the victims' narratives increased across treatment, that the percentage of reported actions and dialogue decreased, and that the percentage of thoughts and feelings increased. In particular, the reported thoughts that attempted to organize and structure the memory of rape substantially increased. This finding indicated that rape victims' narratives of traumatic memories changed over time with the imaginal reliving of the trauma. In particular, the individuals sought to make sense of their memory of the rape and their feelings about that event by structuring their recall in a way that provided a sense of coherence. That sense of coherence may provide a strong feeling of narrative truth and may feel right for both the patient and the therapist, as it were, but it may not provide an unblemished indication of the historical truth of the event, especially given the changes that occur to memory over time (Sarbin 1995; Spence 1982, 1994). The fact that narrative and historical truth may not coincide is nonproblematic and manageable in the clinic by those therapists with relevant knowledge and skill but becomes problematic in nonclinical settings, such as the courtroom, in which the focus of activity and the demands of proof are quite different from those in the clinic (Schutte 1994; Spiegel and Scheflin 1994). As Spiegel and Scheflin (1994) commented, "it is just as possible to dissociate and then retrieve a real memory as it is to convince oneself of a false belief. In the absence of independent corroboration, especially in criminal cases, memory alone cannot fully be trusted" (p. 422).

A number of studies, which have examined whether memories of childhood sexual abuse can be repressed, have raised questions about the trust that can be placed in recovered memory and the utility of such memory in the clinic and in the courtroom (for reviews, see Lindsay and Read 1994; Pope and Hudson 1995). Lindsay and Read (1994) provided a comprehensive analysis of psychotherapy and memory of childhood abuse and argued, in particular, that therapies that involve the recovery of memory can lead to the creation of illusory memories. They focused their comments on memories of abuse that could be said to be the outcome of the use of particular therapeutic techniques, which Lindsay and Read (1994) referred to as "memory recovery therapies." In contrast, Pezdek (1994) argued that the type of memory recovery therapy that was criticized by Lindsay and Read (1994) was not used to a significant degree in psychotherapy and that no clear evidence existed for the creation of illusory memories of sexual abuse by therapists. Pezdek (1994) indicated that many individuals come to therapy with reasonably clear memories of childhood sexual abuse and that other individuals come to therapy after the spontaneous recovery of memory in the absence of any therapeutic intervention. Nevertheless, Banks and Pezdek (1994) considered that "recovered memories can be accurate . . . and compelling memories can be completely unfounded" (p. 267), and these memories may even coexist (Baars and McGovern

1995). Ceci and Loftus (1994) stated that the problem of the creation of illusory memories was pervasive and was not limited to particular individuals or approaches to therapy. They argued strongly that "clients can be led to co-construct vivid memories of events that never transpired; repeated suggestions, imagery instructions, journal writing, and trance inductions are potent psychological mechanisms that we are beginning to realise can lead to false memories" (Ceci and Loftus 1994, p. 362).

Pope and Hudson (1995) reported a detailed analysis of four studies (Briere and Conte 1993; Herman and Schatzow 1987; Loftus et al. 1994b; Williams 1994) and sought to determine whether confirmatory evidence of the abuse had been presented and whether amnesia for the abuse had been demonstrated in these four studies. Note that these were the only relevant studies that Pope and Hudson (1995) could locate, and they concluded that the four studies did not present confirmatory evidence of the abuse and did not demonstrate amnesia for the abuse. Therefore, Pope and Hudson (1995) argued that the "present evidence is insufficient to permit the conclusion that individuals can 'repress' memories of childhood sexual abuse" (p. 126). Notwithstanding this conclusion, it is useful to consider these and other relevant studies for the information that they convey. At the very least, these studies present the difficult conceptual, methodological, and inferential issues that are involved in conducting research on recovered memory of childhood sexual abuse.

In an early study, Herman and Schatzow (1987) reported on the recovered (or suspected) memories of childhood sexual abuse of women who were in group therapy. Because of the problems in understanding the nature of the sample of women, the nature of the memory deficits that they had experienced or were experiencing, the corroboration of abuse claimed by some subjects, and the fact that some cases that were presented by the authors were apparently composites of several cases, it is very difficult to draw meaningful inferences from this study.

More recently, Harvey and Herman (1994) reported on the memories of three adults with childhood trauma. The first case involved the continuous recall of sexual abuse, but with different interpretations and understandings of the events that were said to constitute the abuse; the second case involved a mixture of partial recall and shifts in the individual's understanding of childhood sexual abuse; and the third case involved substantial amnesia by the individual of childhood sexual abuse. Harvey and Herman (1994) highlighted the multiple pathways that can lead to the reporting of memories of childhood sexual abuse in the clinical setting and the different clinical approaches that should be used in these different types of cases. Moreover, they underscored that these different types of cases relate to issues concerning the forensic implications of different pathways to a memory, and they usefully argued that "a science of memory must be able to account for the aberrations of memory and consciousness [and that] effective treatment of these [aberrations] can and must be informed by basic research" (Harvey and Herman 1994, p. 305). Many would agree with this point, but it is difficult to keep it in focus in the politically charged nature of current culture (e.g., Dershowitz 1994; Herman 1995; Hughes 1993; Kaminer 1993; Loftus et al. 1995; Sykes 1992).

In this respect, Briere (1995; see also Brown 1995; Herman 1995) saw limitations with a scientific approach in resolving debate about recovered memory and argued that much of the debate revolved around political issues such as public education, improved professional training, and the marginalization of abuse survivors. Importantly, Briere (1995) highlighted the need for increased attention to standards of professional practice in the area of trauma-oriented psychotherapy, which is a point that needs to be underscored.

Briere and Conte (1993) reported findings from a sample of individuals who were in therapy and indicated that 59% of these patients had identified a period in their lives when they had no memory of the occurrence of childhood molestation. Moreover, the findings suggested that the more violent the abuse and the earlier the abuse occurred, the more likely it was that a period of amnesia had been experienced. Also, the findings indicated that patients who had experienced periods of amnesia had more current psychological symptoms than those who had not. Briere and Conte (1993) acknowledged that their research was limited in several ways, including problems with the selection of their sample (e.g., the individuals were in therapy, and the therapist chose whom to include in the sample) and with the accuracy of the individuals' reports of childhood molestation and periods of amnesia (e.g., they were asked whether there was ever a time when they could not remember an abuse experience). Moreover, it is clear that the corroboration of the patients' reports of childhood sexual abuse was problematic; of course, this is a major issue in this area of research in general (Briere and Conte 1993).

In a somewhat similar study, Loftus et al. (1994b) interviewed women with a history of abuse and asked them whether they had forgotten the abuse for a period of time. Although, and in contrast to Briere and Conte (1993), only 19% of these women indicated such a period, the meaning of this finding is not clear because of the same methodological problems that characterize the study by Briere and Conte (1993). In other research, Elliott and Briere (1995) examined the recall of childhood sexual abuse in a sample of the general population and found that 42% of the respondents with a history of sexual abuse had experienced less memory of the abuse at some time in their life than at other times. Moreover, delayed recall or the recovery of memory was associated with the reported use of threats at the time of the childhood sexual abuse. Finally, those respondents who had recently recovered memories of abuse were reported to have more clinical symptomatology than those who had not. In their focus on a nonclinical sample, Elliott and Briere (1995) importantly suggested the need for a closer examination of the recovery of memory away from the therapeutic setting.

Williams (1994; see also Williams 1995) interviewed women who had histories of sexual abuse in childhood that had been documented in hospital records. She found that 38% of the women did not recall the abuse that had been documented 17 years previously. In particular, those women who were younger at the time of the abuse and those who had been molested by someone they knew were more likely not to recall the previously documented abuse. Given these findings, Williams (1994) argued that the recovery of memories of childhood sexual abuse by some women should not be surprising and that the absence of a memory of abuse should not be seen as necessarily indicating that no abuse occurred during childhood. Loftus et al. (1994a) reviewed and highlighted many of the strengths and weaknesses of this important study. In particular, they indicated how the findings supported the claim that individuals can forget a sexually abusive experience but did not support any claim that childhood sexual abuse is typically set aside from awareness and reliably recovered during adulthood. As Loftus et al. (1994a) noted, some of the women were so young when they were abused that the information was probably not encoded adequately, and others who were abused when older may have simply forgotten the events, as they had forgotten many other events of childhood.

Williams's (1994) research emphasized that some individuals who were sexually abused in childhood may not report such abuse during a clinical examination because they have forgotten it. This study is important not only because it provided information of value and indicated some of the problems involved in conducting meaningful research, but also because the reception and discussion of the findings by both scientists and practitioners interested in this issue indicated how easy it is to mislead and to be misled in this debate (see Loftus et al. 1994a). That is, the complexity of the findings is occasionally masked by overly simplified statements about the inferences that can be drawn from them.

The findings of these various studies underscore that recovered memories of abuse should not be seen as self-validating. Their nature and accuracy must be determined independently rather than being simply assumed by the patient, the therapist, or others. Unfortunately, as Bowers and Farvolden (1996) have stated, "what complicates the situation is that many therapists accept such abuse memories at face value, in part because they feel they are rejecting the patient unless they confirm each and all of his or her ideas, memories, and beliefs" (p. 361). This tendency by some therapists is unfortunate, not only because it may provide the essential approval for the patient to assume the validity of memories that may not be accurate, but also because it conveys that the therapist knows the truth about the patient. For instance, Herman (1992) considered that the "therapist should make clear that the truth is a goal constantly to be striven for, and that while difficult to achieve at first, it will be attained more fully in the course of time" (p. 148). We should recognize, and be comfortable with, the fact that therapists do not know historical truth (Spence 1982, 1994), and to convey otherwise is professional arrogance of the worst kind. As Bowers and Farvolden (1996; see also Lynn and Nash 1994; Lynn et al. 1994) highlighted, "neither the therapist nor the patient has privileged access to the origins of a patient's distress. The therapist can have more or less plausible theories regarding why the patient is distressed, but such theories should not be mistaken for the Truth—however compelling the theory may seem" (p. 373).

Recovered Memory and Well-Being

For some, the recovery of memories of sexual abuse is an essential part of the therapeutic experience and central to the successful outcome of therapy (Courtois 1992, 1995; Olio 1989). For others, the assumption that memories of childhood sexual abuse need to be recovered encourages an attitude of victimization and is counterproductive to the successful outcome of therapy (Loftus et al. 1995; Nash 1994). For instance, Loftus et al. (1995) commented, "[T]herapy that focuses exclusively on the past and what might have been done to the client, still leaves the client wallowing in the victim role. We have only traded one cultural myth for another: that we are never responsible for our own problems or our own healing" (pp. 307–308).

Therapy that focuses on recovered memory may, in fact, have negative effects on well-being. For instance, McElroy and Keck (1995) provided case analyses of three women with eating or obsessive-compulsive disorders who were told that their symptoms were based on childhood sexual abuse and that the recovery of memories of this abuse would be important in treatment. Two of the women were unable to recover any such memories, and their conditions deteriorated; their conditions improved in response to traditional treatment. McElroy and Keck (1995) argued that pressuring patients to recover memories of abuse when they do not believe that they have been abused may have significant negative consequences for treatment. In other work, Byrne and Sheppard (1995) presented 11 case histories of individuals who either made allegations of childhood sexual abuse or had such allegations made against them; in each case, the allegations were either withdrawn or disproved. Based on their analysis of these cases, Byrne and Sheppard (1995) argued for the need for particular guidelines to be developed to identify the possible occurrence of false memory and to treat individuals who are experiencing false memories of childhood sexual abuse.

Brenneis (1994) highlighted how a psychoanalyst who strongly believes in the recovery of early traumatic experiences may make direct and indirect suggestions that will encourage patients to produce false beliefs about such experiences. He indicated that analysts should be aware of the potential risks and benefits of having a strong belief in the possibility of recovering traumatic memories and that the current evidence suggests that the risks to the patient's well-being are likely to be greater than the potential benefits (see also Haakrn 1995). Relatedly, Person and Klar (1994) argued that psychoanalytic notions have blurred distinctions between unconscious fantasies and repressed memories of sexual abuse, and they used a case analysis to discuss problems that psychoanalytically oriented therapists have in dealing with this distinction. Although Person and Klar (1994) argued that memory and fantasy can be disentangled, it must be noted that in the absence of corroboration, little evidence supports the reliability of any such method of differentiation.

In the relevant studies and case reports in the literature, a major issue is the difficulty in obtaining a clear understanding of the "presumed therapeutic benefits of various memory recovery techniques" (Grossman and Pressley 1994, p. 279). No convincing studies or individual cases appear to clearly demonstrate the nature of the benefits that would be derived from the recovery of memory. It may be that techniques do lead to benefit when used by appropriately trained individuals but not by those who are essentially incompetent. There may be value in the recovery of memory if it occurs in the context of genuinely therapeutic activities rather than as a therapeutic activity in its own right. Enns et al. (1995) stated that the experienced and knowledgeable therapist "does not imply that childhood sexual abuse is the only issue that contributes to the client's current psychological status or that this issue must receive greater attention than other issues that the client faces" (p. 229) and also that "major gaps in the client's memory for the past should be noted but the [therapist] should not assume that these gaps necessarily signify a troubled past" (p. 232).

At present, we simply have no convincing evidence that recovered memory leads to improvements in well-being. Thus, as Grossman and Pressley (1994) indicated, the crucial question of whether the potential benefits outweigh the potential costs of attempts to recover memories of childhood sexual abuse cannot be answered at this stage. Read and Lindsay (1994, p. 430) concluded that

> research evidence does not support the idea that a large percentage of clients who have no conscious recollections of childhood sexual abuse

were in fact abused; [that there is] no compelling evidence in support of the idea that therapeutic approaches designed to help clients recover suspected repressed memories are helpful; [and that] there is substantial evidence consistent with the idea that overzealous use of such techniques and ancillary practices may lead some clients who were not abused as children to come to believe that they were abused.

Similarly, and forcefully, Lindsay (1995) emphasized the need to determine whether the recovery of memory is actually associated with positive therapeutic outcomes and concluded that "there is not a single controlled study demonstrating any beneficial effect of therapeutic efforts to recover hidden memories of [child sexual abuse] in clients who report no abuse history, and there is no convincing evidence to support the claim that practitioners can discriminate between clients with no awareness of abuse histories and clients with no abuse histories" (p. 288).

Guidelines for Practice and Directions for Research

The extent to which guidelines for practice are needed depends in part on the degree to which the knowledge and activities of practitioners are at odds with the evidence that is available about recovered memories of childhood sexual abuse. Poole et al. (1995) conducted two surveys of the opinions and practices of therapists in the United States and the United Kingdom concerning psychotherapy and the recovery of memories of childhood sexual abuse. The findings overall raised concerns about the assumptions held and the suggestive approaches used by some therapists when dealing with recovered memory. For instance, the findings indicated that some practitioners believed that they could identify individuals who had been sexually abused, even when those individuals denied such abuse, and that some practitioners used a range of procedures to encourage patients to recover memories of childhood sexual abuse. Notably, some practitioners saw a very wide range of presenting complaints as being associated with childhood sexual abuse. Most respondents considered that it was important to remember abuse for therapy to be effective, but the vast majority also believed that it was possible to develop illusory memories. It is important to acknowledge that most of the respondents to Poole et al.'s (1995) survey indicated that childhood sexual abuse was relevant to only some of their patients, and there was general concern about the possibility of inadvertently leading patients to create false memories or illusory beliefs about childhood sexual abuse.

Because their members need information and because of their responsibility to patients and society more broadly, various organizations have made formal statements or offered formal guidelines about recovered memories of childhood sexual abuse (e.g., American Medical Association 1994; American Psychiatric Association 1993; American Psychological Association 1994; Australian Psychological Society 1994; British Psychological Society 1995; the "Statement on Memories of Sexual Abuse" by the American Psychiatric Association Board of Trustees [1993] appears in the Foreword to Section II in this volume.) After examination of these statements and guidelines, as well as those offered by individuals (e.g., Bloom 1994; Lindsay and Read 1994; Yapko 1994), the particular points of convergence can be summarized as follows:

- Childhood sexual abuse is an unfortunate reality that sometimes has devastating consequences.
- Memory is potentially unreliable, and people can have memories that are not consistent with historical fact.
- Repression should not be rejected as a possibility, but it cannot be accepted without question.
- The presence of particular problems in adulthood cannot be used as a reliable way of inferring that sexual abuse occurred in childhood.
- Therapists should make sure that in attempting to help their patients, they do not do more harm than good; therapists' responsibilities to their patients are best met through an approach of caution and care about the assumptions that they make and the techniques that they use.
- Recovered memories of childhood sexual abuse may or may not be accurate, and independent corroboration is the only way to determine this.
- Therapists should be mindful that different assumptions, procedures, and demands operate in the clinical and legal contexts; professional and ethical responsibilities are best met by avoiding the excessive encouragement or discouragement of reports of childhood sexual abuse.

Of course, knowing how to work effectively in a setting and climate of ambiguity, uncertainty, and demand from patients is one of the most difficult skills that a therapist has to learn, and a strong argument can be made that specific training is needed to help therapists develop and maintain these skills. Moreover, development of comprehensive manuals for the treatment of those who suspect or recover memories of childhood sexual abuse is necessary, and those treatment manuals must be evidence-based and specify best-practice standards (Beutler and Hill 1992; Lindsay and Read 1994). Consistent with this view, Enns et al. (1995) highlighted the need for competent ethical practice and underscored how competent practice must involve a knowledge of memory research; an understanding of trauma, dissociation, and memory loss; and the development of specific intervention skills and practices. Bowers and Farvolden (1996) offered two essential safeguards for therapy that should be heeded regardless of the problem being treated and the technique being used. First, "Do not define the possibility for healing in terms that require the therapist and the patient to understand the latter's problems in the same way" (p. 373). In other words, convey clearly to patients that although you may have a plausible hypothesis about the reasons for their problems, and the strategies for resolving those problems, the patients do not have to necessarily agree with your view. Equally, therapists should not need to accept the reasons given by patients in order to work in a therapeutically effective way with those patients. Second, "Entertain alternative hypotheses to account for the patient's problems, so as not to fixate on one of them" (Bowers and Farvolden 1996, p. 373). In other words, therapists should consider the various reasons that may account for the problems of patients and should ensure that each of these reasons is given appropriate consideration. Therapists should ensure that their reaction to the essential ambiguity of clinical work is not to adopt a position of ultimately indefensible certainty.

Although many researchers and practitioners are striving to understand the issues involved in memory, trauma, and repression, we have a substantial distance to travel before we can agree on what the relevant data are and how to understand the meaning of those data. When faced with finding our way through the maze surrounding the reporting of recovered memories of childhood sexual abuse, the best approach is one that involves a caring application of scientific knowledge. We need to fill the gaps in our knowledge about the processes involved in the reporting of accurate and inaccurate recovered memories, and particular research is needed to understand more about the encoding, storage, and retrieval of memory of trauma (Wolfe 1995). This research should be conducted in the laboratory and in naturalistic settings, and a balanced analysis of the biological, cognitive, and social processes that are involved in such memory is needed. There are also gaps in our knowledge about therapeutic practices that involve the recovery of memory, and particular research is needed to understand more about the ways in which practices may or may not shape the reported recovered memories of patients. Most basic of all, however, we need to move beyond ideology and belief and determine whether therapy that involves the recovery of memory of childhood sexual abuse is effective in improving the well-being of patients.

After reviewing their survey findings, Poole et al. (1995) derived three major issues that research needs to focus on:

1. Whether memory recovery is helpful for patients
2. Criteria to differentiate patients whose adult problems are based in childhood sexual abuse as opposed to other etiology

3. Particular features and influences of different clinical techniques intended to recover memories of childhood sexual abuse

In focusing more specifically on the hypothesis of repression, Pope and Hudson (1995) drew attention to the need for studies that 1) identify individuals whose sexual abuse had been well documented, 2) identify individuals who had experienced sexual abuse after age 5 years, 3) interview these individuals about any history of trauma, and 4) reinterview those individuals who did not comment on the sexual abuse, and ask them about that abuse. According to Pope and Hudson (1995), this type of rigorous methodology is needed to allow meaningful comment to be made about the existence of repression. The comments provided by many in the field about critical research suggest that we need

- Research that more carefully investigates the differences among the memory reports of patients who do not report, forget normally, and repress memories of particular events of childhood
- Systematic case studies of patients who recover memories of childhood sexual abuse where those memories have been independently determined to be accurate
- Systematic case studies of patients who recover memories of childhood sexual abuse where those memories have been independently determined to be inaccurate
- Research that more carefully investigates the differential effects of therapeutic practices that are used to recover memories of particular events of childhood

Primarily, however, research is needed to address the basic question of whether the recovery of memory of particular events of childhood is of genuine therapeutic benefit. To date, no appropriate large-scale research has investigated this issue. For this—and other—research to be conducted, people must work together rather than in opposition; that is, scientists, practitioners, those reporting recovered memories, and those affected by such reports all have to contribute so that we can gather the necessary data.

Conclusion

In some areas of activity, it is difficult to separate the perspectives of the personal and the professional, and that point has been recognized in this debate. Our personal and professional experiences sometimes shape the way in which we frame questions, interpret responses, and practice therapy. We need to recognize, nevertheless, that therapy with patients who report recovered memories of childhood sexual abuse should proceed with an open attitude, a commitment to evidence-based therapy, and a recognition of the experience of patients in a way that conveys the concern and care that is required when dealing with any reports of childhood sexual abuse.

References

American Medical Association: Report of the Council on Scientific Affairs: Memories of childhood abuse. Chicago, IL, American Medical Association, June 1994

American Psychiatric Association Board of Trustees: Statement on memories of sexual abuse. Washington, DC, American Psychiatric Association, December 1993

American Psychological Association: Interim report of the APA working group on investigation of memory of childhood abuse. Washington, DC, American Psychological Association Public Affairs Office, November 1994

Australian Psychological Society: Guidelines relating to the reporting of recovered memories. Melbourne, VIC, Australian Psychological Society, October 1994

Baars BJ, McGovern K: Steps toward healing: false memories and traumagenic amnesia may coexist in vulnerable populations. Consciousness and Cognition 4:68–74, 1995

Banks WP, Pezdek K: The recovered memory/false memory debate. Consciousness and Cognition 3:265–268, 1994

Barnier AJ, McConkey KM: Reports of real and false memories: the relevance of hypnosis, hypnotizability, and context of memory test. J Abnorm Psychol 101:521–527, 1992

Bartlett FC: Remembering: A Study in Experimental and Social Psychology. Cambridge, MA, Cambridge University Press, 1932

Bass E, Davis L: The Courage to Heal: A Guide for Women Survivors of Child Sexual Abuse, 3rd Edition. New York, HarperPerrenial, 1994

Bekerian DA, Goodrich SJ: Telling the truth in the recovered memory debate. Consciousness and Cognition 4:120–124, 1995

Beutler LE, Hill CE: Process and outcome research in the treatment of adult victims of childhood sexual abuse: methodological issues. J Consult Clin Psychol 60:204–212, 1992

Bloom PB: Clinical guidelines in using hypnosis in uncovering memories of sexual abuse: a master class commentary. Int J Clin Exp Hypn 42:173–178, 1994

Blume ES: Secret Survivors: Uncovering Incest and Its Aftereffects in Women. New York, Wiley, 1990

Bower GH: Awareness, the unconscious, and depression: an experimental psychologist's perspective, in Repression and Dissociation: Implications for Personality Theory, Psychopathology, and Health. Edited by Singer JL. Chicago, IL, University of Chicago Press, 1990, pp 209–231

Bowers KS, Farvolden P: Revisiting a century-old Freudian slip—from suggestion disavowed to the truth repressed. Psychol Bull 119:355–380, 1996

Bremner JD, Krystal JH, Southwick SM, et al: Functional neuroanatomical correlates of the effects of stress on memory. J Trauma Stress 8:527–553, 1995

Brenneis CB: Belief and suggestion in the recovery of memories of childhood sexual abuse. J Am Psychoanal Assoc 42:1027–1053, 1994

Briere J: Child abuse, memory, and recall: a commentary. Consciousness and Cognition 4:83–87, 1995

Briere J, Conte J: Self-reported amnesia for abuse in adults molested as children. J Trauma Stress 6:21–31, 1993

British Psychological Society: Recovered Memories. Leicester, UK, British Psychological Society, January 1995

Brown LS: Toward not forgetting: the science and politics of memory. The Counseling Psychologist 23:310–314, 1995

Bryant RA: Fantasy proneness, reported childhood abuse, and the relevance of reported abuse onset. Int J Clin Exp Hypn 43:184–193, 1995

Byrne P, Sheppard N: Allegations of child sexual abuse: delayed reporting and false memory. Irish Journal of Psychological Medicine 12:103–106, 1995

Ceci SJ, Loftus EF: "Memory work": a royal road to false memories? Applied Cognitive Psychology 8:351–364, 1994

Ceci SJ, Huffmann MLC, Smith E, et al: Repeatedly thinking about a non-event: source misattributions among preschoolers. Consciousness and Cognition 3:388–407, 1994a

Ceci SJ, Loftus EF, Leichtman MD, et al: The possible role of source misattributions in the creation of false beliefs among preschoolers. Int J Clin Exp Hypn 42:304–320, 1994b

Cialdini R: Influence: Science and Practice, 3rd Edition. Glenview, IL, HarperCollins, 1993

Cotton P: Biology enters repressed memory fray. JAMA 272:1725–1726, 1994

Courtois CA: The memory retrieval process in incest survivor therapy. Journal of Child Sexual Abuse 1:15–31, 1992

Courtois CA: Scientist-practitioners and the delayed memory controversy: scientific standards and the need for collaboration. The Counseling Psychologist 23:294–299, 1995

Crews F: The verdict on Freud. Psychological Science 7:63–68, 1996

Davis PJ: Repression and the inaccessibility of emotional memories, in Repression and Dissociation: Implications for Personality Theory, Psychopathology, and Health. Edited by Singer JL. Chicago, IL, University of Chicago Press, 1990, pp 387–403

Dawes RM: House of Cards: Psychology and Psychotherapy Built on Myth. New York, Free Press, 1994

Dershowitz AM: The Abuse Excuse. Boston, MA, Little, Brown, 1994

Dobson M, Markham R: Imagery ability and source monitoring: implications for eyewitness memory. Br J Psychol 32:111–118, 1993

Elliott DM, Briere J: Posttraumatic stress associated with delayed recall of sexual abuse: a general population study. J Trauma Stress 8:629–648, 1995

Enns CZ, McNeilly CL, Corkery JM, et al: The debate about delayed memories of child sexual abuse: a feminist perspective. The Counseling Psychologist 23:181–279, 1995

Erdelyi M: Repression: the mechanism and the defense, in Handbook of Mental Control. Edited by Wegner DM, Pennebaker JW. Englewood Cliffs, NJ, Prentice-Hall, 1993, pp 126–148

Femina DD, Yeager CA, Lewis DO: Child abuse: adolescent records vs adult recall. Child Abuse Negl 14:227–231, 1990

Fisher RP, Geiselman RE: Memory Enhancing Techniques for Investigative Interviewing: The Cognitive Interview. Springfield, IL, Charles C Thomas, 1992

Fivush R: Young children's event recall: are memories constructed through discourse? Consciousness and Cognition 3:356–373, 1994

Fivush R, Schwarzmueller A: Say it once again: effects of repeated questions on children's event recall. J Trauma Stress 8:555–580, 1995

Foa EB, Molnar C, Cashman L: Change in rape narratives during exposure therapy for posttraumatic stress disorder. J Trauma Stress 8:675–690, 1995

Fowler C: A pragmatic approach to early childhood memories: shifting the focus from truth to clinical utility. Psychotherapy 31:676–686, 1994

Frankel FH: The concept of flashbacks in historical perspective. Int J Clin Exp Hypn 42:321–336, 1994

Fredrickson R: Repressed Memories: A Journey to Recovery From Sexual Abuse. New York, Simon & Schuster, 1992

Freyd JJ: Betrayal trauma: traumatic amnesia as an adaptive response to childhood abuse. Ethics and Behavior 4:307–329, 1994

Ganaway GK: Transference and countertransference shaping influences on dissociative syndromes, in Dissociation: Clinical and Theoretical Implications. Edited by Lynn SJ, Rhue JW. New York, Guilford, 1994, pp 317–337

Ganaway GK: Hypnosis, childhood trauma, and dissociative identity disorder: toward an integrative theory. Int J Clin Exp Hypn 4:127–144, 1995

Garry M, Loftus EF: Pseudomemories without hypnosis. Int J Clin Exp Hypn 42:363–378, 1994

Garry M, Loftus EF, Brown SW: Memory: a river runs through it. Consciousness and Cognition 3:438–451, 1994

Goldstein E: Confabulations: Creating False Memories—Destroying Families. Boca Raton, FL, SIRS Books, 1992

Goldstein E, Farmer K: True Stories of False Memories. Boca Raton, FL, Upton Books, 1993

Goodman GS, Quas JA, Batterman Faunce JM, et al: Predictors of accurate and inaccurate memories of traumatic events experienced in childhood. Consciousness and Cognition 3:269–294, 1994

Green BL: Introduction to special issue on traumatic memory research. J Trauma Stress 8:501–504, 1995

Grossman LR, Pressley M: Introduction to the special issue on recovery of memories of childhood sexual abuse. Applied Cognitive Psychology 8:277–280, 1994

Haakrn J: The debate over recovered memory of sexual abuse: a feminist-psychoanalytic perspective. Psychiatry: Interpersonal and Biological Processes 58:189–198, 1995

Harvey MR, Herman JL: Amnesia, partial amnesia, and delayed recall among adult survivors of childhood trauma. Consciousness and Cognition 3:295–306, 1994

Herman J: Trauma and Recovery. New York, Basic Books, 1992

Herman JL: Crime and memory. Bull Am Acad Psychiatry Law 23:5–17, 1995

Herman J, Schatzow E: Recovery and verification of memories of childhood sexual trauma. Psychoanalytic Psychology 4:1–14, 1987

Holmes DS: Investigations of repression: differential recall of material experimentally or naturally associated with ego threat. Psychol Bull 81:632–653, 1974

Holmes D: The evidence for repression: an examination of sixty years of research, in Repression and Dissociation: Implications for Personality Theory, Psychopathology, and Health. Edited by Singer JL. Chicago, IL, University of Chicago Press, 1990, pp 85–102

Howe ML, Courage ML, Peterson C: How can I remember if "I" wasn't there: long-term retention of traumatic experiences and emergence of the cognitive self. Consciousness and Cognition 3:327–355, 1994

Hughes R: Culture of Complaint: The Fraying of America. New York, Oxford University Press, 1993

Hyman IE, Husband TH, Billings FJ: False memories of childhood experiences. Applied Cognitive Psychology 9:181–197, 1995

Johnson MK, Raye CL: Reality monitoring. Psychol Rev 88:67–85, 1981

Johnson MK, Hashtroudi S, Lindsay DS: Source monitoring. Psychol Bull 114:3–28, 1993

Kaminer W: I'm Dysfunctional, You're Dysfunctional: The Recovery Movement and Other Self-Help Fashions. New York, Vintage Books, 1993

Kendall-Tackett KA, Williams LM, Finkelhor D: Impact of sexual abuse on children: a review and synthesis of recent empirical studies. Psychol Bull 113:164–180, 1993

Kihlstrom JF: Hypnosis, delayed recall, and the principles of memory. Int J Clin Exp Hypn 42:337–345, 1994

Kihlstrom JF: The trauma-memory argument. Consciousness and Cognition 4:63–67, 1995

Kihlstrom JF, Barnhardt TM: The self-regulation of memory: for better and for worse, with and without hypnosis, in Handbook of Mental Control. Edited by Wegner DM, Pennebaker JW. Englewood Cliffs, NJ, Prentice-Hall, 1993, pp 88–125

Krass J, Kinoshita S, McConkey KM: Hypnotic memory and confident reporting. Applied Cognitive Psychology 2:35–51, 1988

Kuyken W, Brewin CR: Autobiographical memory functioning in depression and reports of early abuse. J Abnorm Psychol 104:585–591, 1995

LeDoux JE: Systems and synapses of emotional memory, in Memory: Organization and Locus of Change. Edited by Squire LR, Weinberger NM, Lynch G, et al. New York, Oxford University Press, 1991, pp 205–216

LeDoux JE, Romanski L, Zagoraris A: Indelibility of subcortical memories. J Cognitive Neuroscience 1:238–243, 1989

Levitt EE, Pinnell CM: Some additional light on the childhood sexual abuse–psychopathology axis. Int J Clin Exp Hypn 43:145–162, 1995

Lindsay DS: Contextualizing and clarifying criticisms of memory work in psychotherapy. Consciousness and Cognition 3:426–437, 1994

Lindsay DS: Beyond backlash: Comments on Enns, McNeilly, Corkery, and Gilbert. The Counseling Psychologist 23:280–289, 1995

Lindsay DS, Read JD: Psychotherapy and memories of childhood sexual abuse: a cognitive perspective. Applied Cognitive Psychology 8:281–338, 1994

Loftus EF: The reality of repressed memories. Am Psychol 48:518–537, 1993

Loftus EF, Ketcham K: The Myth of Repressed Memory: False Memories and Allegations of Sexual Abuse. New York, St Martin's Press, 1994

Loftus EF, Garry M, Feldman J: Forgetting sexual trauma: what does it mean when 38% forget? J Consult Clin Psychol 62:1177–1181, 1994a

Loftus EF, Polonsky S, Fullilove MT: Memories of childhood sexual abuse: remembering and repressing. Psychology of Women Quarterly 18:67–84, 1994b

Loftus EF, Milo EM, Paddock JR: The accidental executioner: why psychotherapy must be informed by science. The Counseling Psychologist 23:300–309, 1995

Lynn SJ, Nash MR: Truth in memory: ramifications for psychotherapy and hypnotherapy. Am J Clin Hypn 36:194–208, 1994

Lynn SJ, Rhue J: Fantasy-proneness: hypnosis, developmental antecedents, and psychopathology. Am Psychol 43:35–44, 1988

Lynn SJ, Rhue J (eds): Dissociation: Clinical and Theoretical Perspectives. New York, Guilford, 1994

Lynn SJ, Myers B, Sivec H: Psychotherapists beliefs, repressed memories of abuse, and hypnosis: what have we really learned? Am J Clin Hypn 36:182–184, 1994

MacLean HN: Once Upon a Time: A True Story of Memory, Murder, and the Law. New York, HarperCollins, 1993

Macmillan M: Freud Evaluated: The Completed Arc. Amsterdam, North-Holland, 1991

Markham R, Hynes L: The effect of vividness of imagery on reality monitoring. Journal of Mental Imagery 17:159–170, 1993

McConkey KM: The effects of hypnotic procedures on remembering: the experimental findings and their implications for forensic hypnosis, in Contemporary Hypnosis Research. Edited by Fromm E, Nash MR. New York, Guilford, 1992, pp 405–426

McConkey KM: Hypnosis, memory, and the ethics of uncertainty. Australian Psychologist 30:1–10, 1995

McConkey KM, Sheehan PW: Hypnosis, Memory, and Behavior in Criminal Investigation. New York, Guilford, 1995

McElroy SL, Keck PE: Misattribution of eating and obsessive-compulsive disorder symptoms to repressed memories of childhood sexual or physical abuse. Biol Psychiatry 37:48–51, 1995

Nachmani G: Trauma and ignorance. Contemporary Psychoanalysis 31:423–450, 1995

Nash MR: Memory distortion and sexual trauma: the problem of false negatives and false positives. Int J Clin Exp Hypn 42:346–362, 1994

Nash MR, Hulsey TL, Sexton MC, et al: Long-term sequelae of childhood sexual abuse: perceived family environment, psychopathology, and dissociation. J Consult Clin Psychol 61:276–283, 1993

Neisser U, Fivush R: The Remembering Self. Cambridge, MA, Cambridge University Press, 1994

Nemiah JC: The unconscious and psychopathology, in The Unconscious Reconsidered. Edited by Bowers KS, Meichenbaum D. New York, Wiley, 1984, pp 49–87

Nogrady H, McConkey KM, Perry C: Enhancing visual memory: trying hypnosis, trying imagination, and trying again. J Abnorm Psychol 94:195–204, 1985

Ofshe RJ, Singer MT: Recovered-memory therapy and robust repression: influence and pseudomemories. Int J Clin Exp Hypn 42:391–410, 1994

Ofshe RJ, Watters E: Making Monsters: False Memories, Psychotherapy, and Sexual Hysteria. New York, Charles Scribner's Sons, 1994

Olio KA: Memory retrieval in the treatment of adult survivors of sexual abuse. Transactional Analysis Journal 19:93–100, 1989

Ornstein PA: Children's long-term retention of salient personal experiences. J Trauma Stress 8:581–605, 1995

Pendergrast MH: Victims of Memory: Incest Accusations and Shattered Lives. Hinesburg, VT, Upper Access Books, 1994

Pennebaker JW, Memon A: Recovered memories in context: thoughts and elaborations on Bowers and Farvolden. Psychol Bull 119:381–385, 1996

Person ES, Klar H: Establishing trauma: the difficulty distinguishing between memories and fantasies. J Am Psychoanal Assoc 42:1055–1081, 1994

Pezdek K: The illusion of illusory memories. Applied Cognitive Psychology 8:339–350, 1994

Poole DA, Lindsay DS, Memon A, et al: Psychotherapy and the recovery of memories of childhood sexual abuse: U.S. and British practitioners' opinions, practices, and experiences. J Consult Clin Psychol 63:426–437, 1995

Pope HG, Hudson JI: Can memories of childhood sexual abuse be repressed? Psychol Med 25:121–126, 1995

Read JD, Lindsay DS: Moving toward a middle ground on the false memory debate: reply to commentaries on Lindsay and Read. Applied Cognitive Psychology 8:407–435, 1994

Roesler TA, McKenzie N: Effects of childhood trauma on psychological functioning in adults sexually abused as children. J Nerv Ment Dis 182:145–150, 1994

Romans SE, Martin JC, Anderson JC, et al: Factors that mediate between child sexual abuse and adult psychological outcome. Psychol Med 25:127–142, 1995

Sarbin TR: A narrative approach to "repressed memories." Journal of Narrative and Life History 5:51–66, 1995

Saywitz KJ, Moan-Hardie S: Reducing the potential for distortion of childhood memories. Consciousness and Cognition 3:408–425, 1994

Schachter DL, Kagan J, Leichtman MD: True and false memories in children and adults: a cognitive neuroscience perspective. Psychology, Public Policy, and Law 1:411–428, 1995

Schooler JW: Seeking the core: the issues and evidence surrounding recovered accounts of sexual trauma. Consciousness and Cognition 3:452–469, 1994

Schulte JG, Dinwiddie SH, Pribor EF, et al: Psychiatric diagnoses of adult male victims of childhood sexual abuse. J Nerv Ment Dis 183:111–113, 1995

Schutte JW: Repressed memory lawsuits: potential verdict predictors. Behavioral Sciences and the Law 12:409–416, 1994

Singer JL (ed): Repression and Dissociation: Implications for Personality Theory, Psychopathology, and Health. Chicago, IL, University of Chicago Press, 1990

Spence DP: Narrative Truth and Historical Truth. New York, WW Norton, 1982

Spence DP: Narrative truth and putative child abuse. Int J Clin Exp Hypn 42:289–303, 1994

Spiegel D (ed): Dissociation: Culture, Mind and Body. Washington, DC, American Psychiatric Press, 1994

Spiegel D, Scheflin AW: Dissociated or fabricated? Psychiatric aspects of repressed memory in criminal and civil cases. Int J Clin Exp Hypn 42:411–432, 1994

Sykes CJ: A Nation of Victims: The Decay of the American Character. New York, St Martin's Press, 1992

Terr L: Unchained Memories: True Stories of Traumatic Memories, Lost and Found. New York, Basic Books, 1994

Tromp S, Koss MP, Figueredo AJ, et al: Are rape memories different? A comparison of rape, other unpleasant, and pleasant memories among employed women. J Trauma Stress 8:607–627, 1995

van der Kolk BA: The body keeps the score: memory and the evolving psychobiology of posttraumatic stress. Harvard Review of Psychiatry 1:253–265, 1994

van der Kolk BA, Fisler R: Dissociation and the fragmentary nature of traumatic memories: overview and exploratory study. J Trauma Stress 8:505–525, 1995 van der Kolk BA, Saporta J: The biological response to psychic trauma: mechanisms and treatment of intrusion and numbing. Anxiety Research 4:199–212, 1991

Walker EA, Gelfand AN, Gelfand MD, et al: Medical and psychiatric symptoms in female gastroenterology clinic patients with histories of sexual victimization. Gen Hosp Psychiatry 17:85–92, 1995

Weinberger DA: The construct validity of the repressive coping style, in Repression and Dissociation: Implications for Personality Theory, Psychopathology, and Health. Edited by Singer JL. Chicago, IL, University of Chicago Press, 1990, pp 337–386

Weingardt KW, Loftus EF, Lindsay DS: Misinformation revisited. Memory and Cognition 23:72–82, 1995

Williams LM: Recall of childhood trauma: a prospective study of women's memories of child sexual abuse. J Consult Clin Psychol 62:1167–1176, 1994

Williams LM: Recovered memories of abuse in women with documented child sexual victimization histories. J Trauma Stress 8:649–674, 1995

Wolfe J: Trauma, traumatic memory, and research: where do we go from here? J Trauma Stress 8:717–725, 1995

Wright L: Remembering Satan. New York, Knopf, 1994

Yapko MD: Suggestions of Abuse: True and False Memories of Childhood Sexual Trauma. New York, Simon & Schuster, 1994

Chapter 8

Intentional Forgetting and Voluntary Thought Suppression: Two Potential Methods for Coping With Childhood Trauma

Wilma Koutstaal, Ph.D., and Daniel L. Schacter, Ph.D.

> My strongest asset through all my experiences was my ability to "block out" whatever I didn't want to remember. If I didn't talk about them, or even think about them, I was able to survive.
>
> *Anonymous incest victim (Silver et al. 1983, p. 97)*

Extreme trauma often evokes equally extreme responses. In the effort to cope, and faced with a life-threatening or world-view shattering traumatic event, an individual may find herself or himself vulnerable to radical alterations in cognitive, emotional, and neurophysiological responses. Posttraumatic stress disorder (PTSD) (e.g., Krystal et al. 1995), psychogenic amnesia (e.g., Schacter et al. 1982), fugue states (e.g., Eisen 1989), and dissociative identity disorder (e.g., Putnam 1993; Schacter et al. 1989) are among such responses. Yet not all individuals respond to trauma with such "extreme" coping mechanisms, nor are all sources of trauma immediately and consistently identified as such. Some forms of trauma, including childhood sexual abuse, may assume a more chronic, ambiguous, and intermittent course, interspersed with periods of comparative normality (see Conte et al. 1989; Trickett and Putnam 1993). What forms of coping might a child attempt to draw on in dealing with such abuse? If abuse is (for the moment) not occurring, and the individual is "expected" to continue with social, familial, and other roles and responsibilities as if nothing had happened, how might the individual attempt to manage thoughts and memory of the abuse?

In this chapter, we specifically focus on two less extreme responses—intentional forgetting and voluntary thought suppression—that represent more commonplace, but potentially important, possible responses to abuse. Although clear evidence supports the role of pro-

---

Preparation of this chapter was supported by National Institute on Aging Grant AG08441.

cesses similar to intentional forgetting and thought suppression in cases of both childhood sexual abuse and adult trauma (and we begin by reviewing some of this evidence), we also attempt to address a further question. What evidence is available from empirical laboratory research that would help us determine when such strategies might or might not prove successful?

We do not assume that intentional forgetting and thought suppression are the only, or even the most important, methods used in coping with sexual abuse or other forms of trauma (although this may be true for some individuals). Equally important, we do not assume that there is evidence for a form of massive and unconscious repression of trauma, in which individuals allegedly become entirely amnesic for repeated or prolonged periods of severe abuse. There is little evidence for such massive repression (see Holmes 1990; Loftus 1993; Ofshe and Singer 1994; Pope and Hudson 1995), and instances of broadly encompassing amnesia may be more likely to involve dissociative pathology than unconscious "repression" (for discussion, see Schacter 1996; Schacter et al., in press; Spiegel 1995). Rather, we are specifically concerned with deliberate and *conscious* efforts at curtailing one's thoughts and memories. We ask: 1) Is there evidence or reason to believe that intentional forgetting and thought suppression are sometimes used (either alone or as a supplement to other methods) in coping with sexual abuse or other forms of trauma? and 2) What does research from laboratory paradigms reveal about the probable effects of these methods on later thinking and memory?

This chapter has four major sections. We begin by briefly reviewing several sources of evidence suggesting that intentional and conscious efforts to suppress one's thoughts and memory of traumatic experiences are, indeed, sometimes used by individuals in attempting to cope with the trauma. In the main part of this chapter, we focus on the empirical literature regarding directed forgetting and thought suppression. In these sections, we assess evidence of the degree to which, and the conditions under which, intentional forgetting and voluntary thought suppression can produce their intended effects. We also provide an assessment of the processes believed to underlie successful intentional forgetting and thought suppression. In the final section, we attempt briefly to interrelate key findings from these two paradigms with clinical and other reports of trauma and suggest several questions that future research should examine.

Evidence Regarding Conscious Efforts to Suppress or to Forget Trauma

Evidence from several sources converges in suggesting that traumatic events—including childhood sexual abuse—may sometimes be followed by deliberate and conscious efforts to suppress thoughts and memories of the abuse. Three general sources of evidence supporting such efforts include

1. Retrospective self-reports obtained during interviews or from questionnaires asking how individuals responded to childhood abuse or other forms of trauma
2. Observations reported by others after a traumatic event, indicating that traumatized individuals sought to avoid reminders or thoughts of the incident or actively denied that it had occurred
3. General background information about the conditions often surrounding revelations of childhood abuse

Excerpts from follow-up interviews recently reported by L. M. Williams (1995) with women who had a documented history of sexual abuse during childhood clearly implicate deliberate and intentional efforts not to think about the abuse as a potential contributor to poor recall of some abuse episodes. In an earlier study, L. M. Williams (1994) found that of 129 women with a documented incident of abuse in childhood, 62% recalled the particular abuse episode that had occurred some 17 years earlier, which had resulted in their being brought to the attention of the investigators. However, additional questioning of these women revealed that not all of them had always remembered the abuse. Of the 75 women who recalled the abuse and who were also asked additional questions, 12 women (16%) reported that there was a time in their past when they had forgotten the abuse—in some cases, after a deliberate and purposeful effort to do so. One woman said, "I blocked it out right away, the first time it happened (age 12). . . . I didn't remember until it happened again—I was raped when I was 17" (p. 663). Two other women used the identical expression of "blocking it out" and further noted how, after a time, they specifically stopped thinking of the abuse: "I don't know how old I was, I used to think about it for the first two years, then I just blocked it out. I may not have completely forgot, I just didn't think about it" (p. 663); "Well I guess I may not have *completely* forgotten about it after my mother talked to me, but blocked it out most of the time, just stopped thinking about it" (p. 666).

These responses are remarkably similar to the efforts at suppression reported by adult rape victims (Burgess and Holmstrom 1979). Some adult victims reported that they attempted to dispel all memory of the rape from their minds through a deliberate and conscious effort. They did not like to be reminded of the rape ("Don't refresh my mind to it") and spoke of being able to "block the thoughts" from their minds (Burgess and Holmstrom 1979, p. 1280). These responses are also similar to that of one woman, anonymously questioned by Silver et al. (1983), about how she had coped with father-daughter incest that had occurred years earlier and who wrote: "My strongest asset through all my experiences was my ability to 'block out' whatever I didn't want to remember. If I didn't talk about them, or even think about them, I was able to survive" (p. 97).

There is also at least some evidence of denial of traumatic events during childhood, soon after those events occurred. For example, in their study of children's memory for an invasive and painful medical procedure (involving urinary tract catheterization), Goodman et al. (1994, p. 288) reported that "a few" of the children from a sample of 46 denied that they had ever undergone the procedure. Likewise, a recently reported and corroborated case of recovered memory for an incident of childhood sexual abuse (Nash 1994) indicated at least *behavioral* denial of the event directly after it occurred.

Children may also actively avoid reminders associated with other forms of trauma. For example, Nader et al. (1990) found that 14 months after a sniper attack on a school playground, of all the children—including those who were on the playground, in the school, or away from the school on that day—66% reported avoidance of reminders of the attack. Of those who were on the playground itself during the attack, nearly 90% still reported avoidance of reminders. In the entire group, avoidance of reminders was the most common symptom still present at 14 months, and the next two most frequently occurring symptoms were fear when thinking of the event (48% of the entire group) and becoming upset by thoughts of the event (47%).

The need or desire to keep abuse secret, either absolutely, so that no one is ever told of the abuse, or selectively, so that only a few trusted others learn of it, may also encourage deliberate efforts at thought suppression and avoidance of reminders that might prompt memories and thoughts of the abuse (see Lane and Wegner 1995). In a national survey of childhood sexual abuse in adult men and women, Finkelhor et al. (1990) found that fewer than 50% of the men and women reporting abuse also reported that they had told anyone about it within a year of its occurrence. Of 169 men who reported a childhood sexual abuse experience, 42% reported that they had never told anyone of the abuse; likewise, of 416 women reporting abuse, 33% indicated that they had never told anyone.

In some cases of childhood abuse, the perpetrator or others who learn of the abuse may actively encourage thought suppression or forgetting by urging secrecy, telling the child that the event never happened, or refusing to discuss the incident (e.g., Adams-Tucker 1982; Browne and Finkelhor 1986; Everson et al. 1989). For example, researchers who have sought to determine the degree of maternal support offered to sexually abused children in clinical samples have found that relatively few mothers are supportive, with the proportion of mothers deemed supportive ranging between 25% and 56% (e.g., Adams-

Tucker 1982; Everson et al. 1989). In a sample of 84 mothers of children with substantiated occurrences of intrafamilial sexual abuse, Everson et al. (1989) found that only 44% of the mothers provided consistent support during the period following disclosure of the abuse (e.g., made clear and public statements of belief in their child, or actively demonstrated disapproval of the perpetrator's abusive behavior). An additional 32% provided ambivalent or inconsistent support (e.g., wavered in believing the child, or remained passive, refusing to take sides), and 24% were unsupportive or rejecting of their children (e.g., were threatening or hostile, or totally denied that the abuse occurred).

Based on questionnaire results anonymously asking a large (non-clinical) sample of women how they had attempted to make sense of their earlier experiences of father-daughter incest, Silver et al. (1983, p. 97) concluded that "the ability to block or interrupt thoughts of a negative event may be crucial in living with events that have, in fact, no resolution." Based on her interviews with women with documented instances of abuse, L. M. Williams (1995, p. 668) concluded that "forgetting about the child sexual abuse is for some a motivated, volitional forgetting (in a conscious attempt to deal with the abuse by blocking it out)."

Deliberate and conscious efforts to minimize thinking about an abusive episode or to purposefully block it from awareness may—at least in some instances—provide an immediate means of coping with the abuse. Do such efforts also reduce the ease and likelihood that the abuse will be remembered?

Evidence accumulated across decades of experimental research on memory has shown that the more a stimulus or event is cognitively elaborated on and interassociated with other aspects of one's knowledge, the more likely it is that the stimulus or event will be remembered (e.g., Craik and Tulving 1975; Fivush and Schwarzmueller 1995; Tessler and Nelson 1994; for review, see Schacter 1996). Research on the degree to which individuals can forget when instructed or "directed" to do so points to a similar conclusion. However, research on directed forgetting has also emphasized other factors that may—sometimes quite substantially—alter the likelihood and ease with which events will be accessed. Prominent among these factors are aspects of the *retrieval environment* in which memory is probed, including both the degree to which item-specific cues are present (i.e., features or aspects similar to the to-be-remembered event or stimulus itself) and the degree to which the more general environmental and cognitive context of the individual corresponds to that present during the initial encounter with the material (for review and discussion, see Davies and Thomson 1988; Koutstaal and Schacter, in press). Intriguingly, the physical and mental circumstances present during an individual's efforts to suppress a particular thought have also emerged as prominent considerations in the experimental work on voluntary thought suppression, influencing the likelihood that suppression will be successful or will lead to the exact *opposite* of the hoped-for result: greater rather than diminished preoccupation with the unwanted thought.

We next review findings from these two laboratory paradigms. In each case, we first examine basic outcome data on the degree to which the intended outcome (forgetting or reduced frequency of the unwanted thought) can be achieved and then consider possible mechanisms underlying those effects. We examine experiments using both emotionally neutral and emotionally significant materials; in addition, in the case of directed forgetting, we also briefly consider studies that investigated whether children can intentionally forget.

Intentional Forgetting

Can Adults Intentionally Forget Emotionally Neutral Materials?

Clear and consistent experimental evidence indicates that instructing an individual to forget something can subsequently result in diminished memory for that material compared with memory for information that was never subjected to an intention to forget (for reviews, see Bjork 1989; H. M. Johnson 1994). However, whether intentional forgetting will be successful depends on a variety of factors relating both to the conditions present during the encoding of the to-be-forgotten information and to the conditions under which retrieval is attempted.

One factor that has emerged as particularly important in determining the extent to which memory for the to-be-forgotten items is, indeed, impaired relative to memory for items that were designated as to-be-remembered concerns the manner in which the instruction to forget is given. Two methods of providing the instruction to forget have been most frequently explored by cognitive researchers in recent years. In one method, individuals are first presented an entire set or block of items under intentional learning conditions. They are then unexpectedly told that this information should be forgotten—usually under the guise that the first block of items were "practice" items. In this method—hereafter referred to as the "block-cuing" directed forgetting procedure—the instruction to forget is given only after subjects have already encountered and actively attempted to remember many stimuli. In contrast, in a second method, individuals are told at the outset that the experiment is concerned with how well people can selectively remember some information while forgetting other information. In this method—hereafter referred to as the "item-cuing" directed forgetting procedure—each stimulus item is designated either as to-be-remembered or as to-be-forgotten soon after it is presented (usually within a few seconds).

The second of these methods, in which some of the stimulus items are cued as to-be-forgotten soon after they are encountered, generally results in more forgetting than in the first method, in which the instruction to forget is postponed until after a larger set of items has been presented. Table 8–1 presents a comparison of the amount of forgetting observed on free- or cued-recall tests with the item-cuing versus block-cuing procedure. Results are shown for eight experiments or experimental conditions in which both of these cuing procedures were used within the same experimental design (Basden et al. 1993a, 1994; Koutstaal 1996). As can be seen in Table 8–1, both procedures resulted in greater recall of the remember-cued than the forget-cued items. However, the differences were consistently larger in the item-cuing than in the block-cuing procedure, resulting in an average difference of 27% for the item-cuing (range, 14%–45%) compared with only 12% for the block-cuing method (range, 6%–21%).

With the item-cuing procedure, forgetting is also generally found during recognition testing (e.g., Bjork and Geiselman 1978; Golding et al. 1994). In contrast, the strong retrieval cues provided by the recognition test items usually eliminate the disadvantage for the forget-cued

Table 8–1. Magnitude of directed forgetting on recall tests under item cuing and block cuing

Experiment and type of test	Item cuing			Block cuing		
	Rem	For	Diff	Rem	For	Diff
Basden et al. (1993a)						
Expt. 1 cued recall	.35	.14	.21	.33	.24	.09
Expt. 2 cued recall	.82	.59	.23	.74	.65	.09
Expt. 3 free recall	.50	.05	.45	.41	.20	.21
Expt. 4 free recall,						
short list	.25	.11	.14	.33	.22	.11
Expt. 4 free recall,						
long list	.23	.08	.15	.19	.10	.09
Basden et al. (1994)						
Expt. 1 free recall	.53	.12	.41	.44	.24	.20
Koutstaal (1996)						
Expt. 4 free recall	.37	.12	.25	.35	.24	.11
Expt. 5 free recall	.42	.07	.35	.34	.28	.06
Average directed						
forgetting effect			.27			.12

Note. All results are for the first test administered only.
Rem = remember cued; For = forget cued; Diff = difference in remember-cued and forget-cued performance (Rem – For).

items under block cuing (e.g., Basden et al. 1993a, 1994; Geiselman et al. 1983; Koutstaal 1996, Experiments 3 and 4). Table 8–2 presents the outcome of 12 experiments that used the item-cuing method, in which subjects were tested by using recognition, and in which recognition was the first test administered. In these experiments, the average directed forgetting effect was 18% (range, 7%–35%). In contrast, a set of 8 experiments that used the block-cuing method yielded an average directed forgetting effect of only 2% (range, –2%–9%).

Do these differences in memory performance for the to-be-remembered versus the to-be-forgotten items arise from *impaired* memory for the *forget-cued* items? Or do they primarily reflect *enhanced* memory for the *remember-cued* items? As will be seen, comparisons of the data provided in Tables 8–1 and 8–2 as well as other sources of evidence suggest that the answer to this question depends on the method that is em-

Table 8–2.   Magnitude of directed forgetting on recognition tests under item cuing and block cuing

Experiment and condition	Item cuing			Block cuing		
	Rem	For	Diff	Rem	For	Diff
Basden et al. (1993a)						
Expt. 1	.88	.77	.11	.92	.89	.03
Expt. 2	.92	.77	.15	.90	.89	.01
Expt. 4, short list	.81	.67	.14	.86	.88	−.02
Expt. 4, long list	.75	.59	.16	.76	.74	.02
Basden et al. (1994)						
Expt. 1	.86	.67	.19	.89	.83	.06
Koutstaal (1996)						
Expt. 1	.86	.67	.19	—	—	—
Expt. 2	.94	.87	.07	—	—	—
Expt. 3	—	—	—	.98	.97	.01
Expt. 4	.89	.70	.19	.85	.86	−.01
Expt. 5	.93	.58	.35	.87	.78	.09
Gardiner et al. (1994)						
Short cue delay	.68	.43	.25	—	—	—
Long cue delay	.67	.55	.12	—	—	—
MacLeod (1989)						
Expt. 1, immediate test	.76	.55	.21	—	—	—
Average directed forgetting effect			.18			.02

Note.   All results are for the first test administered only. Dashes indicate that the relevant procedure (item cuing or block cuing) was not included in a particular experiment and condition.

Rem = remember cued; For = forget cued; Diff = difference in remember-cued and forget-cued performance (Rem − For).

ployed. Whereas the differences found in the item-cuing procedure may primarily result from preferentially thinking about and elaborating on the remember-cued items, this account does not seem to apply as well to the forgetting observed in the block-cuing procedure. With block cuing, the to-be-forgotten items may be less readily retrieved from memory *despite* having been initially processed and encoded to the same degree as the to-be-remembered items. However, further discussion of the possible processes underlying directed forgetting will be postponed until evidence regarding forgetting of emotionally significant materials and directed forgetting in children has been examined. At this point, however, we can draw five conclusions from the above discussion and from the data provided in Tables 8–1 and 8–2 concerning the forgetting of emotionally neutral material:

1. There is clear evidence that the intention to forget certain experimentally presented materials can lead to reduced memory performance for those items compared with stimuli that were not subjected to an intention to forget.
2. Under conditions of relatively little retrieval support (such as during free-recall or cued-recall testing), the decrease in memory for the forget-cued items has been observed both when individual items are cued as to-be-forgotten soon after their presentation (item cuing) and when the instruction to forget is given only after several stimuli have already been actively processed (block cuing).
3. Under conditions of greater retrieval support (such as recognition testing), the decrease in memory for the forget-cued items has most often been seen only under item cuing and not with block cuing.
4. Despite the presence of sometimes quite substantial differences in memory performance for the to-be-remembered and to-be-forgotten items, *some* of the to-be-forgotten items are still recalled and recognized. For example, the average level of recall for the forget-cued items in Table 8–1 was 16% under item cuing and 27% under block cuing; likewise, the average level of recognition for the forget-cued items in Table 8–2 was 65% under item cuing. Thus, directed forgetting seems to involve a relative rather than absolute phenomenon.
5. The directed forgetting effects obtained with item cuing tend to be greater than those found with block cuing and are also greater under free- or cued-recall test conditions than under recognition testing. The latter observation is important because it partially addresses the concern that directed forgetting effects are simply due to voluntary response withholding—that is, a failure to report information about the to-be-forgotten items even though that information is, in fact, remembered. If individuals were merely fail-

ing to report the to-be-forgotten items, it is not clear why they would more often fail to report that information during one testing situation (e.g., under recall testing) than another (e.g., recognition testing; see, for example, Brandt et al. 1985; Spanos et al. 1990; Williamsen et al. 1965; see also Schacter 1986).

Can Adults Intentionally Forget Emotional or Traumatic Stimuli?

The findings concerning intentional forgetting of emotional materials are somewhat mixed but, on the whole, indicate that forgetting can also occur for emotionally significant materials, at least under some circumstances. Two studies have specifically reported failures to forget emotionally negative materials or a failure to forget either emotionally negative or emotionally positive materials. In one study (Geiselman and Panting 1985, Experiment 2), undergraduate students were presented a list of words, one-half of which were judged to be positive in meaning (e.g., clown, butterfly, love) and one-half of which were judged to be negative in meaning (e.g., garbage, disease, dirt). The item-cuing method was used, with the positive and negative words presented in intermixed fashion for 3 seconds each, and immediately followed by an instruction either to remember or to forget (also for 3 seconds). Analyses of subjects' free-recall responses revealed a significant interaction of cue type with word affect, indicating that for the remember-cued items, positive words were significantly more likely to be recalled (mean, 64%) than negative words (mean, 43%), but the reverse was true for the forget-cued items; when given an instruction to forget, negative words were significantly more likely to be recalled (mean, 31%) than were positive words (mean, 16%).

More recently, Ochsner and Schacter (unpublished observations, February 1996) used a modified block-cuing procedure to determine whether recollection of emotionally charged photographs could be affected by intentional forgetting. Subjects were instructed to either remember or forget six-item blocks of photographs that depicted scenes and objects with neutral emotional content (e.g., a rolling pin or an office scene), positive content (e.g., a happy family), or negative content (e.g., a mutilated limb). All items in a given block were of the same emotional valence. On a subsequent recognition test, when subjects indicated that an item was old (i.e., was previously presented in the experiment), they were asked to indicate whether they could also "recollect" particular details regarding the photograph's prior occurrence, such as its appearance or their reaction to it, or whether they simply "knew" that the item had been previously presented, without being able to recollect any specific episodic details about it. (For a general review of this procedure, known as the *remember/know* distinction but

---

here referred to as *recollect/know* so as to avoid confusion with the instruction cue, which is also designated as *remember*, see Gardiner and Java 1993.) The key finding was that directed forgetting affected only memory for neutral items. In general, negative photographs produced the most, and neutral photographs the fewest, recollections, but when subjects were instructed to forget, recollections of negative and positive items were unchanged, whereas recollections of neutral items were reduced by 40%.

This study suggests that, under certain conditions, both positive and negative emotional information may be resistant to conscious attempts to forget. However, three other studies have yielded either more mixed conclusions or evidence of successful forgetting of emotionally significant materials. Using the block-cued directed forgetting procedure, Myers et al. (1992) found no effect of emotional valence on the recall of words. In this study, a manipulation of the valence of the words (positive, negative, or neutral) was combined with another individual differences factor. The subjects (female undergraduate students) were classified on the basis of their performance on the Marlowe-Crowne Social Desirability Scale (Crowne and Marlowe 1964) and the short version of the Taylor Manifest Anxiety Scale (Taylor 1953) into four groups: 1) repressors (high defensiveness and low anxiety, $n = 15$), 2) low anxious (low defensiveness and low anxiety, $n = 15$), 3) high anxious (low defensiveness and high anxiety, $n = 12$), and 4) defensive high anxious (high defensiveness and high anxiety, $n = 12$) (for the original development of this classification scheme, see Weinberger et al. 1979). Two blocks of items, each composed of six positive, six negative, and six neutral words, were presented. Subjects were required to rate each of the words for pleasantness and then were told, after the first block, that those items were for practice and could be forgotten. Averaging across the groups, there was significant directed forgetting (average recall of to-be-remembered items, 32%; average recall of to-be-forgotten items, 19%). However, there was no interaction of group with instruction cue, indicating that the magnitude of the directed forgetting effect was similar for all four subject groups. Also, although there were too few observations for the differently valenced words to be analyzed separately, examination of the mean number of to-be-forgotten words that were recalled showed no evidence that negative words were either more or less likely to be forgotten than positive or neutral words (average recall of to-be-forgotten negative, positive, and neutral words of 9%, 7%, and 3%, respectively; average recall of to-be-remembered negative, positive, and neutral words of 11%, 13%, and 8%, respectively).

Using a quite different procedure, in which individuals were administered shocks for retrieving to-be-forgotten items, Weiner (1968, Experiments 6, 7, and 8) found that individuals were modestly but significantly less likely to retrieve information when they knew they would be shocked for doing so (average recall across three experiments, 55%) than when no shock would follow on retrieval (average recall, 60%). Although the investigators attempted to ensure that these differences were not simply due to voluntary response withholding, this alternative cannot be definitively ruled out.

The most directly relevant study to address the issue of directed forgetting and trauma arising from childhood sexual abuse is that of McNally et al. (unpublished observations, February 1996). These investigators used the item-cuing procedure to examine the extent to which women who had been sexually abused as children could selectively remember or forget trauma-related words (e.g., molested, scream), positive words (e.g., healthy, secure), and neutral words (e.g., curtain, desk). Performance was examined separately for those women who had a current diagnosis of PTSD ($n = 14$) and those who did not currently have PTSD ($n = 12$). The words (10 from each category) were presented in intermixed fashion, with each word presented for 2 seconds, followed by the instruction cue to remember or to forget for 3 seconds. All subjects were tested first on free recall, then on cued recall (the recall cues consisted of the first three letters of each word), and finally on a yes/no recognition test (composed of the 30 studied items and 30 new nonstudied distractor items, with the distractor items also being drawn from the trauma-related, positive, and neutral categories).

In the PTSD participants, although memory for the trauma-related words was greater with an instruction to remember (38%) than with an instruction to forget (26%), the overall level of recall of the trauma-related words (32%) significantly exceeded that for the positive and neutral words (mean, 15%), which were entirely unaffected by the instruction cue (mean for remember cue, 15%; mean for forget cue, 15%). PTSD participants recalled significantly fewer positive to-be-remembered words (11%) and significantly fewer neutral to-be-remembered words (19%) than did control participants (29% and 45%, respectively). In contrast, the non-PTSD participants recalled a similar number of trauma-related and non-trauma-related words overall and had better memory for the to-be-remembered items than for the to-be-forgotten items, regardless of the valence of the words (to-be-remembered recall for trauma-related, positive, and neutral words of 33%, 29%, and 45%, respectively; to-be-forgotten recall for the same categories, respectively, of 23%, 15%, and 20%). A very similar pattern was found in cued recall. The PTSD participants tended to recall more of the trauma-related words (54% remember, 48% forget) than the neutral or positive words (average, 28%), and this trend was largely unaffected by the instruction, whereas the non-PTSD control subjects showed overall directed forgetting. On the recognition test, PTSD participants recognized significantly fewer of the to-be-remembered words than did the control subjects; also, whereas PTSD participants showed no overall directed forgetting in recognition, the non-PTSD control subjects again showed directed forgetting.

On the one hand, considering the participants with PTSD, this study indicates a *failure* of selective forgetting of trauma-related material: these participants tended to remember trauma-related words that they were supposed to forget and failed to remember non-trauma-related words that they were supposed to remember. On the other hand, considering the participants who did not have PTSD, this study also suggests that successful intentional forgetting of trauma-related material is possible. Despite having a history of childhood abuse, the non-PTSD participants *were* able to selectively remember and to forget, with that ability manifested for both the trauma-related items and non-trauma-related items.

Extrapolation of these findings to settings outside the laboratory must be done cautiously. The ability to selectively remember or forget the presentation of single word cues in an experimental setting—even words semantically associated with a form of trauma that an individual experienced—is clearly not equivalent to the ability to remember or forget the trauma itself or even the environmental and other cues actually associated with the trauma. Furthermore, in themselves, these results cannot explain why PTSD participants were less able to forget trauma-related words than were their non-PTSD counterparts who had also endured childhood abuse. For example, did PTSD participants have more extensive and more strongly activated general schemata for abuse, thus making it both more difficult to forget the trauma-related words and more difficult to remember the non-trauma-related words? Nonetheless, these results suggest that the effectiveness of intentional forgetting of abusive episodes might be moderated by factors relating to the psychological status of the individual at the time. Voluntary forgetting of trauma-related materials may not be possible for some individuals (e.g., those with PTSD) but may be possible for others (e.g., those without PTSD). Other factors, possibly correlated with the presence or absence of PTSD, such as the severity or nature of the abuse, may, of course, also be important.

Can Children Show Intentional Forgetting?

Is intentional forgetting possible for young children? Because many incidents of abuse occur during childhood, this question is clearly important.

Four studies have examined children's ability to forget neutral materials (Bray et al. 1983, 1985; Harnishfeger and Pope 1996; Howard and

Goldin 1979), and each demonstrated that children may—under certain conditions—be able to successfully attend to, and remember, relevant rather than irrelevant information. However, if the information is designated as to-be-forgotten only after the child has already encountered it, then younger children (kindergarten children; 7-year-olds; and, to a lesser degree, 9-year-olds) prove largely unable to selectively forget.

Three of these studies used a somewhat different directed forgetting procedure, in which each child was presented with several trials, but some trials included an instruction to forget some of the items. Howard and Goldin (1979) showed kindergarten children (mean age, 5.8 years) a female doll, named "Amy," who (they explained) had to wear special items of clothing to signal that she was a secret agent. The child's task was to help Amy remember which items were special on any one day (i.e., experimental trial). This task was challenging because the items were always drawn from a set of 16 items, including 1 of 4 different hats (e.g., the hat could be a pillbox, beret, ski cap, or sailor hat), 1 of 4 different belts, 4 colors of flowers, and 4 types of neckpieces. Both the number of items that were said to be part of the "special signal" and the number of items that were presented but were not (for that trial) part of the special signal were varied across trials.

The investigators found that children could very efficiently selectively encode relevant information if they were told what types of items (e.g., hat and belt) were relevant *before* the doll was presented. In this case, children showed little interference from the presentation of other (but currently irrelevant) items. However, if children were told what types of items were relevant only after encoding, then they showed interference from the irrelevant items that were also presented.

Using a design in which children were repeatedly presented with one or two sets of pictures, but were sometimes told to forget one of the sets, Bray et al. (1983) also found that the youngest children (age 7 years) had no enhancement in the ability to remember the to-be-remembered items because the other items were cued as to-be-forgotten. For these children, performance was the same as if the child had been presented with both sets of items and was asked to remember both sets. However, 9-year-old children showed some ability to benefit from the forget cue, yet not as much as 11-year-olds, who showed complete elimination of the interference from the forget-cued items. (The latter result was also obtained with 11-year-olds in a subsequent study by Bray et al. 1985 and is also found with adults.)

More recently, the block-cuing directed forgetting procedure typically used with adults has also been studied in children. Harnishfeger and Pope (1996, Experiment 1) presented children (first-, third-, and fifth-graders) with a list of 20 unrelated words, with directions to repeat each word out loud as it occurred and to try to remember it. The children were interrupted after the first 10 words and were told either that the words presented up to that point had been "for practice" and so should be forgotten or that they should continue to remember the words while the next half of the list was presented. On a subsequent free-recall test, the fifth-graders (mean age, 11.5 years) showed consistent and significant directed forgetting, third-graders (mean age, 9.5 years) showed directed forgetting on one measure but not another (forgetting in a within-subjects comparison but not in a between-subjects comparison), and first-graders (mean age, 7.2 years) showed no directed forgetting. An essentially similar pattern was obtained in a replication study (Harnishfeger and Pope 1996, Experiment 2) that included an additional manipulation check to ensure that the children understood the directions given to them at the midpoint of the study list.

What do these findings imply about the ability of children to selectively encode—or remember—information in situations outside the laboratory, particularly situations involving abuse? Any form of direct extrapolation of these findings to such situations is clearly impossible. Nonetheless, they suggest that although even relatively young children may have the capacity to channel their efforts at remembering—provided that they know, at the outset, what it is that they are to try to remember—younger children may be less able to selectively forget information that they have already encoded and processed. By early adolescence, however, children may also be able to selectively forget stimuli or events even after that information has been encoded, effectively exercising control over information already present in memory rather than only precluding entry of information into memory in the first place.

What Processes Underlie Successful Intentional Forgetting?

Three processes have been postulated to underlie the successful forgetting of to-be-forgotten information that has been observed in the laboratory:

1. *Selective search of the to-be-remembered items*, according to which individuals are thought to initially code or "tag" to-be-remembered stimuli differently from to-be-forgotten stimuli and, then, during attempted retrieval, to somehow limit their search for a given item only to the to-be-remembered items
2. *Preferential encoding and rehearsal of the to-be-remembered stimuli*, according to which individuals more extensively process the to-be-remembered items than the to-be-forgotten items
3. *Retrieval inhibition*, according to which the intention to forget initiates a form of suppression such that the to-be-forgotten items are rendered less accessible during retrieval than the to-be-remembered items (Other processes that might render retrieval more dif-

ficult but that do not necessarily involve "inhibition" in a strict sense are also possible.)

Evidence supportive of a possible role for each of these processes has been found.

The strongest evidence for a contribution of selective search to successful forgetting has been obtained using a multitrial short-term memory procedure (e.g., Epstein and Wilder 1972; Homa and Spieker 1974; Howard 1976) that differs in several ways from the item-cuing and block-cuing directed forgetting procedures described earlier in this chapter. Although selective search may also contribute to enhanced memory for the to-be-remembered items under the block-cuing procedure (particularly when only the to-be-remembered items are tested), it does not seem sufficient to account for the full pattern of results under either that procedure or the item-cuing procedure. For example, it is not clear why—provided that individuals *know* that the to-be-forgotten items are being probed—memory for the to-be-forgotten items should be impaired. Why can individuals not just broaden their memory search to include both the to-be-remembered and the to-be-forgotten items?

Recent work has thus focused on evaluating the likely contribution of the second and third processes: preferential encoding of the to-be-remembered items on the one hand and disrupted access to the forget-cued items during retrieval on the other. The preponderance of the evidence suggests that intentional forgetting under the item-cuing method derives from more elaborative and extensive encoding of the remember-cued items. In contrast, several sources of evidence suggest that a form of inhibition or disruption of retrieval access is most likely involved in the block-cuing procedure.

The differential pattern of forgetting on recall versus recognition testing is perhaps one of the more important sources of data supporting this distinction. A pattern of impaired access to information during recall testing combined with intact performance during recognition testing has long been thought to indicate that the information must have been *available* in memory (or how could it have been recognized?) but for some reason was *inaccessible* during attempted recall (Tulving and Pearlstone 1966). Conversely, impaired performance despite the presence of strong and specific retrieval cues, such as those provided by a recognition test, has been thought to point to the possibility that the nonrecognized items were not stored in the first place (i.e., were not only inaccessible but also unavailable) (e.g., Roediger and Crowder 1972). Important caveats apply to this general rule (e.g., under certain conditions, the content or structure of the recognition test itself may make it more difficult to access information that is available in memory); nonetheless, impaired memory for the to-be-forgotten items during recognition testing under the item-cuing method—but not under the block-cuing method—is highly consistent with the notion that the to-be-forgotten items may have an encoding disadvantage with the former but not the latter method.

A comparison of the task demands under the two methods also supports the plausibility of this interpretation. On the one hand, the close proximity of the instruction cues to the initial presentation of the stimulus items under the item-cuing procedure leaves ample room for subjects to adopt a "wait-and-see" approach in their efforts to comply with the task. That is, before making a full-scale effort to remember a given item, subjects involved in the item-cuing procedure might "wait and see" if the instruction cue indicates that the item is, indeed, supposed to be remembered, fully elaborating on and actively rehearsing only those items that are subsequently cued as to-be-remembered and minimally processing the forget-cued items. On the other hand, the postponement of the forget instruction under the block-cuing procedure until many items have been processed and subjects' initial unawareness that a forget instruction will be given at all both suggest that these items were initially adequately encoded and processed but subsequently rendered less accessible.

Two further findings are consistent with the interpretation that the forget-cued items are less extensively elaborated on under item cuing but not under block cuing: 1) subjects' recollection for the forget-cued items is strongly impaired in item cuing but either not impaired or only minimally impaired in block cuing, and 2) conceptual priming for the forget-cued items may be reduced in item cuing but not block cuing. Subjects' memory for the to-be-forgotten items when they are instructed to remember or to forget on an item-by-item basis is much less often accompanied by additional information about the internal or external circumstances under which they first encountered the items than is true for the to-be-remembered items. Asked to indicate not only whether they recognize previously presented stimuli but also whether they can recollect any specific episodic details about their earlier encounter with the stimulus (e.g., what the item led them to think about), subjects involved in the item-cuing procedure had a very poor recollection of the items they were instructed to forget (Basden et al. 1993b; Gardiner et al. 1994; Koutstaal 1996; for a general review and description of this remember/know procedure, see Gardiner and Java 1993). In contrast, when subjects were instructed to forget using the block-cuing procedure, recollection of the circumstances surrounding the forget-cued items either was not impaired (Basden et al. 1993b) or was only slightly diminished, with a significant effect apparent only in a meta-analysis combining results across experiments (Koutstaal 1996). Likewise, recent reports suggesting diminished performance for forget-cued compared with remember-cued items on conceptual implicit tests, including word association (Basden et al. 1993b) and general knowledge questions (Basden and Basden, in press), with the item-cuing procedure but not the block-cuing procedure suggest that in item cuing but not block cuing, the to-be-forgotten stimuli are less elaboratively encoded and processed than the to-be-remembered stimuli. (For discussion of the distinction between perceptual and conceptual implicit tests, see, for example, Roediger et al. 1989; Schacter 1994.)

Nonetheless, it is possible that not *all* of the effects observed with the item-cuing procedure arise from enhanced encoding of the remember-cued items. For example, evidence also indicates that instructing subjects to use a more active form of forgetting—by mentally repeating "STOP" whenever a forget-cued item is presented—enhances the degree of forgetting observed compared with that observed for other strategies, including trying to think of nothing (i.e., trying to make one's mind "go blank") or deliberately rehearsing the to-be-remembered items (Geiselman et al. 1985, Experiment 2). Intriguingly, this enhancement of forgetting as a result of the use of the more active forgetting strategy was apparent only during free-recall testing. Although, overall, both recall and recognition of the to-be-remembered items were greater than that for the to-be-forgotten items, the more pronounced directed forgetting effect due to the use of the "STOP" procedure was apparent only on the recall test. A further experiment indicated that mentally repeating a nonsense word ("DAX") whenever a to-be-forgotten item was presented was less effective in reducing recall than was repetition of the conceptually more meaningful word "STOP" (Geiselman et al. 1985, Experiment 3). These findings suggest that under some conditions, the directed forgetting effect observed with the item-cuing method may also derive, in part, from depressed availability of the forget-cued items (as well as, or in addition to, enhanced memory for the remember-cued items) and that more specific and focused voluntary efforts at suppressing the to-be-forgotten material may more strongly impair memory.

If the intentional forgetting observed under the block-cuing procedure primarily involves a form of suppression or disruption in retrieval access to the to-be-forgotten items, rather than poorer initial storage or encoding, how—more specifically—might such disruption or inhibition "work"? For example, can any other indications of disrupted access be obtained, apart from the diminished ability to recall the items themselves? Although the precise nature of the processes involved is unclear, several findings suggest that the inhibitory or disruptive effects may be somewhat diffuse, encompassing not only the information that was specifically subjected to an intention to forget but also other stimuli or attributes that were associated with the to-be-forgotten information.

Initial evidence suggesting that the instruction to forget might result in diminished access to the entire episode to which the forget instruction was applied was reported by Geiselman et al. (1983). In a series of experiments, they found that subjects who were instructed to forget the first of two blocks of items not only were less likely to recall the items that were designated as to-be-forgotten but also were less likely to recall other incidentally learned items that had been interspersed among the to-be-forgotten items but were never specifically mentioned as a target for forgetting. This diffuse form of forgetting was also observed, at least under some conditions, by Barnhardt (1993) after controlling for a potential artifact in the Geiselman et al. (1983) study and may be similar to a diffuse form of forgetting recently reported by Allen et al. (1995) with hypnotic virtuosos. Allen et al. found that hypnotic virtuosos had posthypnotic recognition amnesia not only for a studied word list for which amnesia was explicitly suggested but also for a word list that was learned during the same hypnotic session but was not covered by any amnesia suggestion—again suggesting that intentional forgetting may assume a more general or broadly encompassing form than is strictly required by the instruction.

Geiselman et al. (1983) noted that subjects who were instructed to forget the first block of items were especially inaccurate at determining when those items had occurred. The order in which subjects recalled the forget-cued items (as well as the incidentally learned items that had been interspersed with those items) also tended to be only weakly correlated with the order in which the items had originally been presented. This was not true for the remember-cued items or for the first block of items in a control group asked to remember the first block. These findings of both relatively poor source memory for the forget-cued items (indicated by difficulties in determining when they had occurred) and impaired retrieval organization for those items (indicated by the tendency to recall the to-be-forgotten items in an order that had little relation to the order in which they had originally been encountered) suggested that access to the forget-cued items might be impeded because of a disruption in the association between the items and representations of the context in which they had been learned.

A recent experiment conducted in our laboratory (Koutstaal 1996) also found evidence of disrupted access to a form of contextual information concerning the forget-cued items. This experiment involved a manipulation that heightened the distinctiveness of the to-be-forgotten versus the to-be-remembered items by associating all of the forget-cued items with one contextual factor (one group of people read all of these items) and all of the remember-cued items with another contextual factor (a different group of people read all of these items). Subjects were significantly less accurate at identifying the group of people who had been associated with the forget-cued items than they were at determining the group of people who had been associated with the remember-cued items. Furthermore, and unlike nearly all previous experiments using block cuing, in this experiment (Experiment 5 in Table 8–2), directed forgetting was also observed during recognition testing.

The observation of impaired memory for the to-be-forgotten items even when retrieval cues were provided suggests that the intentional forgetting of entire episodes of previously encountered information might be facilitated if the to-be-forgotten episode is accompanied by contextual features that differentiate it from other experiences. Differentiating contextual features may allow the to-be-forgotten information to be more efficiently isolated from other information in memory and thus allow more selective forgetting. Contextual change may reduce the frequency with which external reminders of the to-be-forgotten information are encountered. Changes in context may also lead to more internal and possibly largely automatic processes wherein other information, goals, and intentions accompanying the to-be-forgotten information are more effectively deactivated (see Beckmann 1994; Goschke and Kuhl 1993) after environmental and cognitive change than in their absence. Additional research in this direction involving the manipulation of other forms of contextual features (e.g., mood state and general environmental characteristics, such as the place where information is learned) would allow assessment of the possibility that stronger and less readily reversed forgetting of entire episodes may occur if the contexts for the to-be-remembered and to-be-forgotten episodes are sufficiently distinctive.

Nonetheless, although manipulations of context might facilitate forgetting, we reiterate that these effects of intentional forgetting—when observed—involve relative rather than absolute differences. Memory for the to-be-forgotten materials may be diminished relative to memory for the to-be-remembered materials, but a considerable proportion of the to-be-forgotten information is still remembered, with greater memory generally apparent with more adequate retrieval support. Furthermore, although findings concerning directed forgetting have begun to be extended to emotional materials and, in some circumstances, directed forgetting has been observed for emotionally significant materials, this has not been consistently found, and definite counterexamples, with both item-cuing and a modified block-cuing procedure, have also been reported. Thus, whereas, on the whole, the evidence reviewed about intentional forgetting does point to processes that permit restricted encoding and to some extent diminished accessibility of information, these findings provide no evidence supporting the possibility that individuals' conscious attempts to forget will result in massive and complete amnesia for severely traumatizing events.

Voluntary Thought Suppression

The question of whether individuals can intentionally forget information about stimuli or events that they have already encountered and processed is closely linked with another question: To what extent can individuals successfully avoid or suppress conscious thoughts about an unwanted topic (independently of the effects this may have on memory)? Although some investigators have noted the connections between directed forgetting and thought suppression (e.g., Barnhardt 1993; H. M. Johnson 1994; Wegner et al. 1987), several differences in the experimental procedures used to study intentional forgetting and thought suppression have also been identified. Perhaps most important, investigations of voluntary thought suppression have typically involved instructions to suppress thoughts about a single topic or episode, whereas investigations of directed forgetting have most often involved instructions to forget many items of information that are usually entirely unrelated to one another or that are derived from several different semantic categories. (Note that for the block-cuing directed forgetting method, even though an entire set of previously encountered items is designated as to-be-forgotten—and so in one sense a single temporal episode is targeted for forgetting—many different and usually semantically unrelated items are in the block. This differs from having only a single topic or theme to be suppressed.)

Several experiments have investigated the degree to which individuals could successfully suppress thoughts about essentially neutral or innocuous topics. Specifically introduced by the experimenter as a target for attempted thought suppression, these topics have included both relatively whimsical and novel subjects (e.g., thoughts about a white bear or a story about a green rabbit) and more familiar and mundane matters (e.g., thoughts about vehicles or the Statue of Liberty). Can individuals successfully suppress such thoughts? What might experimental investigations of the suppression of such thoughts reveal about the suppression of more emotionally significant and personally relevant topics?

On the one hand, the processes involved in the suppression of thoughts that have considerable emotional and personal significance may well differ in important ways from the processes that allow the eradication or reduced frequency of more neutral thoughts. Emotionally neutral and experimenter-provided thoughts may differ from personally relevant thoughts in how familiar, how complex, and how easily imagined they are and in how much experience individuals have in attempting to control them (Kelly and Kahn 1994). Also, as Salkovskis and Campbell (1994) observed, the emotional effects of the intrusive thoughts may modify the ways in which such thoughts are processed (emotion may affect the nature of the thought itself), and the individual's cognitive appraisal of the meaning and implications of the thoughts may affect the intensity or nature of the motivation to suppress (i.e., thoughts about the thought may influence further affect and motivation about the thought).

On the other hand, exploration of the relative success with which individuals can suppress emotionally neutral or experimentally suggested thoughts allows greater experimental control than is otherwise possible. Such exploration may permit the isolation and identification of factors that may also moderate the suppression of personally relevant thoughts but that—given the idiosyncratic and often complex set of conditions involved in their formation and maintenance—may be very difficult to disentangle. Confining experimental examination of thought suppression to only those thoughts that individuals find intrusive and personally distressing in their lives clearly has its own hazards, not the least of which is sampling bias. When only thoughts that have been identified as intrusive and as recurrent sources of distress are used as objects of experimental investigation, whether (or how often) other thoughts have been successfully suppressed and what conditions allowed such suppression cannot be determined. Ascertaining how, when, and to what extent individuals are able to suppress comparatively unfamiliar and externally introduced thoughts may provide a "window" on the very early processes that are involved in suppression, allowing determination of the conditions that may lead *either* to a future and chronic course of unsuccessful suppression or to successful suppression.

Fortunately, investigators do not need to choose between these two alternatives, and several recent experiments have been reported using targets for suppression that have greater emotional and personal significance to the individuals. We next review some of the central findings from these investigations, beginning with emotionally neutral materials.

Can Adults Voluntarily Suppress Emotionally Neutral Thoughts?

Most of the evidence from studies using emotionally neutral materials indicates at least some degree of *initial* success in suppressing a target thought—when success is measured on the order of several minutes. For example, in one of the earliest studies of thought suppression, Wegner et al. (1987, Experiment 1) compared two groups of subjects. Both groups of subjects first participated in a 5-minute practice session with a stream-of-consciousness technique in which they were asked to verbalize continually what they were presently thinking, without attempting to explain or justify their thoughts. Then, one group of subjects—the *initial suppression* condition—was instructed to continue to verbalize their thoughts in the same manner as before with one important exception: subjects were told, "This time, try not to think of a white bear. Every time you say 'white bear' or have 'white bear' come to mind, please ring the bell on the table before you." Another group of subjects—the *initial expression* condition—were given similar instructions but, instead, were told to "try to think of a white bear." The results showed that the suppression instruction clearly reduced the frequency with which the target thought occurred. After combining all three possible ways in which thoughts of white bears might be indicated (bell ring plus verbal mention of a bear, bell ring only, and verbal mention only), subjects in the initial expression condition had an average of 16.38 overtly indicated thoughts of bears during the 5-minute period. In contrast, subjects in the initial suppression condition had only 6.3 such thoughts. Furthermore, most of these thoughts occurred during the first 2 minutes of the suppression period, such that by the end of 5 minutes, subjects in the suppression condition were overtly indicating fewer than 1 "unwanted" thought per minute.

Most other investigations (e.g., Clark et al. 1991; Wegner et al. 1990, 1991; Wenzlaff et al. 1991) have also found that subjects initially instructed to try to suppress a neutral thought are relatively—albeit not absolutely—successful in doing so. (Note that although the suppression instructions decreased the frequency of the target thought in the study described above, a number of such thoughts still occurred.) Successful suppression has also been observed in comparison to what may be a more natural "think of anything" baseline condition, in which subjects are not asked to express the target thought but instead are instructed to think of anything they like, including the target (Clark et al. 1991, 1993). For example, Clark et al. (1993) compared how often subjects thought about a tape-recorded story about a green rabbit that they had just heard when instructed to suppress all thoughts of the story ("Keep from your mind thoughts of anything that you heard on tape. . . . It is absolutely essential that you try to suppress this material from your mind") with subjects who were instructed to think of anything they wished, including the story ("Think about absolutely anything, with no restrictions, including material you heard on the tape"). Although some 46% of the thoughts verbalized by subjects in the think of anything condition referred to the tape, only 19% of the thoughts verbalized by subjects in the suppression condition referred to the taped material. Individuals in the suppression condition also provided lower ratings than did individuals in the think of anything condition when asked to subjectively rate the amount of time they had spent thinking about the tape. (For two cases in which suppression was not evident in either the expression or the think of anything condition, see, respectively, Muris et al. 1992, 1993.)

However, most of these studies also indicate a further phenomenon that provides an important qualification. Individuals who are first asked to suppress a neutral thought often show a "rebound" in the frequency with which the target thoughts occur, such that during a subsequent postsuppression period, they more often think of the thought than if they had not been asked to suppress. Individuals who earlier tried to suppress a neutral thought and were later either asked to express the thought (e.g., Kelly and Kahn 1994; Wegner et al. 1987, 1991) or were encouraged to think about anything they liked (Clark et al. 1991, 1993) showed significantly more frequent occurrences of the thought than did persons who were never asked to suppress the thought (but were first asked either to express the thought or to think about anything).

Why does this rebound effect occur? Is a resurgence of the frequency of the "unwanted" thought inevitable, or might rebound somehow be prevented, so that voluntary thought suppression would prove to be a more enduring remedy for unwanted thoughts? Most important, does a similar effect occur with emotionally and personally significant materials?

Two primary accounts of the rebound effect have been proposed, each of which has received some support. However, we discuss these accounts—and what the evidence concerning them tells us about the conditions under which successful thought suppression may occur—after a review of studies involving the suppression of emotional materials. Surprisingly, the evidence for rebound effects with emotional materials is considerably less strong than for neutral materials.

Can Adults Voluntarily Suppress Emotionally Significant and Personally Relevant Thoughts?

The findings as to whether adults can voluntarily suppress thoughts that are more intimately associated with their emotional, motivational, and personal lives are decidedly mixed and complex. Both the somewhat equivocal nature of the findings and the complexity arise from three factors: 1) variability in how particular thoughts were selected as targets for suppression, 2) differences in how long (and in what contexts) suppression instructions were maintained, and 3) differences in the characteristics of the individuals chosen for inclusion in the studies.

Unsuccessful suppression, involving a failure to suppress negative or aversive materials, has been reported by several investigators. Two such reports involved instructions to suppress a target thought over a period of several days—including contexts outside the laboratory setting. Muris and Merckelbach (1991, cited in Muris et al. 1992) first read subjects a transcription of Freud's Ratman obsession and then instructed one-half of the subjects to suppress all thoughts of the transcription; the remaining subjects were given no instructions about suppression. One week later, subjects were interviewed as to the frequency with which they had thought of the transcription over the past week. Subjects who had been given suppression instructions reported more intrusions of the thought than did subjects who had not been encouraged to suppress.

Although suggestive, the reliance on individuals' subjective and retrospective reports to determine thought occurrences in this study is clearly highly problematic. A more convincing indication that individuals' longer-term efforts at deliberately suppressing negative thoughts may prove unsuccessful has recently been reported by Trinder and Salkovskis (1994). Subjects in this study (undergraduates) were preselected from a larger population on the basis of a questionnaire describing and assessing negative intrusive thoughts; to be selected into the study, subjects had to report having experienced such thoughts during the preceding month. Individuals who met this criterion were then interviewed on two occasions, separated by 4 days. During the first session, subjects were asked to identify, and then evaluate, a specific negative intrusive thought on various dimensions (e.g., amount of discomfort experienced during the thought). They were also given a habituation sequence for the thought, in which they were repeatedly asked to imagine the thought as clearly as possible and then (again) to evaluate various aspects of the thought. Thereafter, they were assigned to one of three groups: 1) a suppression group, instructed to try to suppress the thought as quickly as possible whenever it came to mind; 2) a control group, instructed simply to record any occurrences of the target thought ("record only" group); or 3) a third group, instructed to think about the target thought as much as possible whenever it occurred without modifying the thought ("think through" group). Subjects were also given postcards on which to write any occurrences of the thought, with separate sections for each of the 4 days, and were given a distinctive reminder cue to wear on their watches to help them remember to record any target thoughts.

Subjects who were asked to suppress experienced *more* of the target thoughts than did subjects in either the record only group or the think through group, which did not differ from each other. Nonetheless, subjects' self-ratings of the degree to which they had attempted to suppress thoughts were higher for the suppression group than for the other groups, suggesting that greater frequency of the target thought occurred despite greater efforts at suppression.

Do these findings indicate that emotional materials cannot be suppressed and that suppression may even lead to precisely the opposite effect—increased rather than decreased cognitive and emotional involvement with the unwanted thought? In answering this question with regard to this study and other studies that have explored thought suppression of emotional materials, it is critical to keep in mind a point raised earlier in this chapter: When only thoughts that have been identified as intrusive and as recurrent sources of distress are used as objects of experimental investigation, whether (or how often) other thoughts have been successfully suppressed and what conditions allowed such suppression cannot be determined. Two forms of "selection bias" may operate in such cases: bias in the *thoughts* within individuals that are selected for examination and bias in the particular *persons* who are selected for the study. For example, in the Trinder and Salkovskis (1994) study, only slightly more than one-half (56%) of the larger population of students that was originally sampled reported having negative intrusive thoughts during the preceding month, and all of the subjects included in the study were selected from this subset of students. What about the other 44% of the sample? Why had they not experienced (or at least not reported having experienced) such thoughts? How might these individuals respond differently to negative or aversive thoughts than the 56% included in the study?

The experimental evidence on thought suppression may be examined with different questions in mind. To investigate whether thought suppression provides a viable model for the occurrence of ruminative or obsessive thinking, selection on the basis of the presence of intrusive and recurrent negative thoughts may well increase ecological validity. But to examine whether individuals—in general—can voluntarily suppress negative or aversive thoughts, preselection of subjects may prove misleading.

It is important that several additional studies that have reported unsuccessful attempts at thought suppression also preselected subjects (e.g., Mathews and Milroy 1994; Salkovskis and Campbell 1994). In contrast, of five studies that either reported successful initial suppression of emotionally significant or negative thoughts (Kelly and Kahn 1994; Roemer and Borkovec 1994; Wegner and Gold 1995; Wegner et al. 1990) or were ambiguous (Muris et al. 1992), none preselected subjects specifically on the basis of intrusiveness or nonintrusiveness of thoughts. Although in two cases, subjects were selected or assigned to particular experimental groups on the basis of the nature and intensity of emotional responses they had to particular situations or persons (Roemer and Borkovec 1994; Wegner and Gold 1995), subjects were not included precisely on the basis of the intrusiveness of particular target thoughts in any of these studies.

Muris et al. (1992) asked subjects (undergraduates) to read a story that involved a highly negative event (subjects were asked to imagine themselves being late for an appointment, speeding through a yellow traffic light, and causing an accident in which a child is killed) or a very similar story in which the emotional words and phrases were replaced by neutral elements. Thereafter, subjects in the emotional and neutral story conditions were assigned either to a suppression condition or to a "think of anything" condition, in which they were free to think or not to think about the story they had read. This first phase, which lasted for 5 minutes, was followed by two 5-minute "think of anything" phases, with the first free expression phase occurring immediately after the initial suppression or expression phase and the second occurring after a 20-minute unrelated task. (Thus, for both the emotional story and the neutral story, one group of subjects received a suppression phase immediately followed by a think of anything phase, followed 20 minutes later by an additional think of anything phase; another group of subjects received a think of anything phase on all three occasions.) During each of the three critical phases, subjects were told to press the button of a hand-held event marker each time they happened to think of the story.

There was no indication that subjects given the suppression instructions—for either the emotional or the neutral story—were successful in less often thinking about the story. Both of these groups tended to think about the story as often as subjects in the emotional think of anything condition, and all of these groups thought of the story more often than subjects in the neutral think of anything condition. In the former three groups (suppress–neutral, suppress–emotional, think of anything–emotional), there was a slight trend for fewer thoughts to occur during the second (think of anything) phase than during the initial phase, and thoughts of the story had clearly decreased by the third (think of anything) phase. On the one hand, the equivalence of the two suppression groups to the think of anything–emotional group during the initial phase does point to a failure of initial suppression. On the other hand, the largely parallel *decrease* in thoughts of the story in all three groups across the later two periods appears to indicate a form of habituation to thoughts of the story over time. Such habituation is clearly inconsistent with the notion that rebound would occur after attempted suppression.

Four studies, using quite different emotional topics as targets for suppression, have provided evidence for successful initial suppression of emotional thoughts. Wegner et al. (1990) examined mentions of target thoughts under suppression compared with expression instructions for an exciting topic (e.g., thoughts about sex) and a relatively less exciting topic (e.g., thoughts about dancing). Although suppression did not entirely eliminate the target thought, mentions were clearly less frequent during suppression than during expression instructions. Evidence also indicated that the frequency of the target thoughts decreased with both suppression and expression instructions for shorter- (4-minute) and longer-term (30-minute) periods, suggesting that thoughts about exciting topics were not especially susceptible to rebound.

Initially successful suppression has also been reported for thoughts about an "old flame" (i.e., a "significant past romantic relationship") (Wegner and Gold 1995), individuals' own intrusive thoughts (Kelly and Kahn 1994), and personal situations specifically associated with depression or anxiety (Roemer and Borkovec 1994). For example, Roemer and Borkovec (1994) found that the proportion of direct statements related to a to-be-suppressed topic situation under initial suppression instructions was 19% for a depressing situation, 26% for an anxious situation, and 17% for a neutral situation; under initial expression instructions, the corresponding proportions were 89%, 67%, and 45%. Suppression was also successful when negative affect statements were the dependent measure, such that under expression conditions, depressed and anxious groups expressed more negative affect than the neutral group, and under suppression instructions, negative affect for the depressed and anxious groups did not differ from that for the neutral group. However, suppression was not observed for *indirect* statements about the situation (e.g., if the subject's depression involved the loss of a friend, but the subject referred to some other loss); such indirect thoughts were not affected by the suppression instruction.

Little evidence of a rebound effect was found in the study by Kelly and Kahn (1994) involving subjects' own intrusive thoughts. In the study by Wegner and Gold (1995), a rebound effect was observed only for participants who suppressed thoughts about an individual they no longer desired or often thought about (a "cold flame"). Whereas cold flame participants reported more thoughts about the past romantic relationship if they had just suppressed thoughts of that relationship than if they had just suppressed thoughts about a neutral topic (e.g., thoughts about the Statue of Liberty), "hot flame" participants, when invited to talk about their past romantic relationship, often spoke about their old flame regardless of whether they had just suppressed thoughts of the flame or had just suppressed thoughts about a neutral topic. Thus, although both hot and cold flame participants were able to initially suppress thoughts about their past romantic relationships, this suppression bore no special costs of increased thinking about the relationship for the hot flame participants, but it did for cold flame participants. (A possible account of this result is provided in the final section.)

In summary, most studies with neutral stimuli indicate some degree of success in *initially* suppressing the target thought. Similar results have been obtained in most studies with more emotionally significant materials—*provided* that subjects were not preselected on the basis of their inability to suppress particular thoughts. However, especially in the case of neutral thoughts, but less so for emotionally significant thoughts, initial suppression is often followed by a rebound. When later given the opportunity either to specifically express the target thought or to think of anything at all, individuals who had earlier suppressed a neutral thought are especially likely to think of that very thought. What might account for this effect, and, equally important, why might it less frequently occur with emotionally significant materials?

What Processes Underlie Successful—and Unsuccessful—Voluntary Thought Suppression?

Analysis of subjects' reported thoughts during their attempts to suppress an unwanted thought revealed that many individuals were using an unfocused form of self-distraction. In their effort not to think about the "forbidden" thought, subjects often focused their attention on various apparently harmless aspects of their immediate surroundings (e.g., the wall, the light switch, their shoes). However, because subjects often focused on these environmental details immediately after they had failed to suppress the unwanted thought, these "would-be distractors" may have become associatively linked with the to-be-suppressed thought—and so may later act as *reminders* of the to-be-avoided topic.

Indirect support for this "association" hypothesis (Wegner and Gold 1995; Wegner et al. 1987) has been obtained from two sources. First, individuals have been found to show more resistance to a rebound of the unwanted thought if they are instructed to use a specific distractor thought. Rather than engaging in an unfocused and haphazard search for satisfactory alternative thoughts in which sundry things may—unwittingly—become cues to the thought, individuals may be encouraged to consistently replace unwanted thoughts with another specific thought. Rebound has been reduced in the presence of focused distraction both with a neutral target (e.g., thoughts of a white bear) as the to-be-suppressed item (Wegner et al. 1987) and with naturally occurring intrusive thoughts. Providing subjects with a specific distractor task to perform during their attempts to suppress a naturally occurring intrusive thought (Salkovskis and Campbell 1994) diminished the frequency with which intrusions occurred, both compared with a condition in which only general (unfocused) distraction instructions were given and compared with the usual suppression instructions (in which no distraction strategies are specifically mentioned). (Interestingly, the clinical use of thought suppression may involve both thought-stopping and instruction in the use of a pleasant distractor thought. See, for example, Kumar and Wilkinson 1971; Turner et al. 1983.)

Although consistent with the association hypothesis, these findings have alternative interpretations. For example, to the extent that reliance on a specific distractor thought results in fewer occurrences of the unwanted thought, then the unwanted thought is itself less elaborated and richly encoded. Less elaborated and richly encoded thoughts may themselves be less readily recalled independent of whether particular cues were associated with the thoughts to prompt their return.

Possibly stronger support for the association hypothesis derives from comparisons of the degree to which individuals are successful in maintaining thought suppression when they are either in an environment that closely matches that in which they initially tried to suppress an unwanted thought or in a situation that differs in important ways. Several studies have found that intrusions of an unwanted thought are less common after the individual's environment is altered, both when external features of the environment are changed and when the individual's mood or "mental context" (Lockhart 1988; Smith 1995) is changed. For example, Wegner et al. (1991) manipulated the external context that was present during thought suppression by showing color slides drawn from different themes (e.g., landscapes or household appliances) during subjects' efforts to suppress thoughts about a white bear and then by showing slides from the same theme or a different theme during a subsequent expression period. The rebound effect was considerably stronger if the slides during initial suppression and later expression were the same than if they were different. There was also evidence that the slides themselves were mentioned more frequently during initial suppression than initial expression instructions (i.e., at the point at which distraction was first occurring), and, during subsequent expression, references to the slides were more often directly followed by references to the white bear for initial suppression than for initial expression subjects.

During unfocused attempts at distraction, individuals may turn their attention not only to various aspects of the external environment but also to their current concerns, intentions, memories, and so forth. To the extent that these internal sources of distraction are filtered by the individual's present mood (e.g., such that depressed people tend to choose negative thoughts as distractors more than do nondepressed people), then altering an individual's mood might act in a manner similar to altering the external environment. By reducing the likelihood that previous distractor *thoughts* return to mind, alterations in an individual's mood should also reduce the likelihood that the *associations* between these earlier thoughts and the unwanted thought will prompt return of the unwanted thought. Alterations in mood have, indeed, been found to act in this way. For example, Wenzlaff et al. (1991) used a mood induction procedure to encourage ("induce") subjects to feel either relatively more or less positive during an initial suppression period and either more or less positive during a later expression period. Although initial suppression subjects showed a rebound effect regardless of whether their mood was the same or different between the earlier and later periods, the rebound effect was stronger if the subjects' mood was congruent in both phases (negative-negative, positive-positive) than if it was incongruent (negative-positive, positive-negative).

This effect was found for suppression of a neutral thought (i.e., thoughts of a white bear). Heightened rebound effects under mood-congruent conditions have also been established with positive and negative autobiographical events, both when mood was experimentally manipulated via a mood induction procedure (Howell and Conway 1992, Experiment 1) and when subjects were assigned to positive and negative mood conditions on the basis of their scores on a self-report measure (Beck Depression Inventory; Howell and Conway 1992, Experiment 2). Wenzlaff et al. (1988) reported that depressed individuals had an especially pronounced rebound effect during the latter part of a 9-minute suppression period if they were asked to suppress thoughts about a highly negative life-event description. Additional analyses of the emotional valence of subjects' thoughts immediately preceding and following negative thought intrusions indicated that nondepressed subjects' thoughts were significantly more positive after the intrusion of a negative target thought than before the thought, but the valence of the thoughts of the depressed subjects did not change. Thus, the nondepressed subjects tended to distract themselves from the negative target thought by focusing on a positive thought, whereas the depressed subjects turned from the negative target thought toward other negative thoughts—ultimately, a less effective strategy.

All of these findings regarding the effects of altered external and internal context on the effectiveness of suppression and the likelihood of rebound are clearly consistent with the association hypothesis. Nonetheless, evidence also suggests that the association hypothesis cannot explain all of the effects (or countereffects!) of suppression. Although diminished in magnitude, rebound effects have also been observed when the context has been different from the original suppression context (Wegner et al. 1991) and with an indirect measure that did not require conscious recollection of the stimulus (Macrae et al. 1994).

Based on these and several additional findings, investigators have proposed an alternative explanation for suppression: the "accessibility" hypothesis. The accessibility hypothesis suggests that rebound occurs because of an "ironic" and automatic mental process (Wegner 1994; Wegner et al. 1993) that is established during the initial intention to suppress. According to the accessibility hypothesis, in addition to suppression per se, successful suppression requires remembering the thought to be suppressed. Whereas suppression involves voluntary or "controlled" cognitive processes in which the individual expends cognitive effort in searching for and maintaining suitable distractor thoughts, remembering what is to be suppressed is an automatic process—a process that operates largely outside of awareness, with little conscious guidance beyond that involved in initiating suppression (e.g., Hasher and Zacks 1979; see Uleman 1989). This involves a constant vigilant monitoring for any occurrences of the to-be-suppressed thought—or of thoughts even remotely or weakly associated with it—so as to quickly suppress the unwanted thought. However, paradoxically, this second automatic process, because it renders the individual unusually attuned to internal and external stimuli associated with the unwanted thought, increases the likelihood that the thought will recur—even with very little prompting or cuing.

If both a controlled process of suppression and an automatic process of detecting stimuli associated with the unwanted thought are occurring, then a manipulation that interferes with the ability to consciously suppress should "uncover" the automatic process. More specifically, if the intention to suppress engenders an automatic process of hypervigilance for items associated with the unwanted thought, then—provided one can effectively circumvent or undermine conscious efforts at suppression through distraction—it might be possible to observe *hyperaccessibility* of the to-be-suppressed thought. Individuals instructed to suppress a target thought might show that thought (and possibly thoughts associated with it) to be even more accessible to them than to individuals who are deliberately attempting to concentrate on that same thought (concentration presumably requiring vigilance but not necessarily hypervigilance).

Consistent with this expectation, Wegner and Erber (1992) found that subjects who were attempting to suppress a particular neutral target thought (e.g., house or mountain) when placed under high "cognitive load" showed hyperaccessibility of the thought. Asked to very rapidly produce associations to various words, subjects who were attempting to suppress a given target word were more likely to give that word as an association than were subjects who were trying to concentrate on the word. Asked to perform the same task but without any particular time pressure, the reverse occurred: subjects concentrating on the topic more often provided it as a response than did subjects suppressing the topic. Additional evidence supportive of altered accessibility of the target thought has also been reported with a modified version of the Stroop task (Wegner and Erber 1992, Experiment 2; see Lavy and van den Hout 1994).

Taken together, all of these findings suggest that both associative cuing and alterations in the accessibility of the target thought may influence the likelihood of successful suppression. As suggested by Macrae et al. (1994), the accessibility hypothesis possibly can be extended or modified to include associative cuing factors. To the extent that features of one's internal or external context become associated with the to-be-suppressed target thought, then the target may receive additional activation when the context is maintained or reinstated. A modified account such as this might also more readily accommodate the findings that reinstatement effects (e.g., Davies and Thomson 1988) and reduced proactive and retroactive interference due to altered contexts (e.g., Kanak and Stevens 1992) may be observed in other paradigms even when no particular conscious or deliberate attention has been directed toward aspects of the environment. We next discuss the possible relevance of these findings and previously reviewed findings on directed forgetting in regard to traumatic situations.

Integration and Relation to Abuse Literature

Our comments in this section focus on three factors: 1) the importance of external and internal context as a moderating factor in both intentional forgetting and thought suppression, 2) the interconnectedness of intentional forgetting and thought suppression with other factors (including other forms of coping) that may affect memory, and 3) future directions and questions.

The Importance of External and Internal Context

The critical role of the amount of retrieval support offered by the environment during attempts to probe memory has long been recognized (e.g., McGeoch 1932; Tulving 1983). However, a review of findings on both intentional forgetting and voluntary thought suppression suggests that retrieval cues may assume a more than usually potent role in prompting the return of to-be-forgotten or to-be-suppressed thoughts. Encountering all (Basden et al. 1993a, 1994; Geiselman et al. 1983; Koutstaal 1996) or even only a few (Bjork and Bjork 1991; Goernert and Larson 1994) of the to-be-forgotten items following an attempt to forget an entire set or block of items may largely eliminate the mnemonic disadvantage for the forget-cued items that would otherwise have been observed. Such "release from retrieval inhibition" (Basden et al. 1993a; Bjork 1989) on reexposure to the to-be-forgotten stimuli is similar to the effect produced by encountering aspects of the environment that were present during earlier attempts at thought suppression. Rebound of thoughts is especially strong in external and internal conditions that closely parallel those prevailing during initial attempts at suppression.

These findings suggest that retrieval cues may also be especially important in prompting the reemergence of thoughts or memories of traumatic incidents when people attempt to suppress or forget those incidents. Many investigators have specifically pointed to the role of retrieval cues in prompting recall of previously forgotten or suppressed incidents of abuse (e.g., Feldman-Summers and Pope 1994) or have reported individual cases consistent with such a view (McNally et al., unpublished data, February 1996; Schooler 1994; see also Christenson et al. 1981; McGee 1984). For example, some anonymous women who were self-reported survivors of father-daughter incest that had occurred an average of 20 years earlier still reported recurrent, intrusive, and disruptive memories, and most respondents reported that memories, thoughts, and images of the experience were likely to be triggered by salient cues in their everyday interactions (Silver et al. 1983).

As the time from an original episode of abuse increases, an individual's external context is likely to have changed, thus increasing the likelihood of successful forgetting. Individuals may also deliberately alter their living or work circumstances to facilitate forgetting. Interviews of adults who had been raped 4–6 years earlier (Burgess and Holmstrom 1979) revealed several strategies that the victims used to cope with the rape. In addition to thought suppression, many individuals changed their residence or traveled. Some victims moved into a new apartment within the same neighborhood, others moved to a completely different neighborhood, and still others (often those with less financial independence) temporarily stayed with relatives or friends. Some of these individuals directly remarked on the positive aspects of moving. For example, one victim said, "I think it was easier for me because I went to another city and wasn't reminded of it. I didn't have to see it every day. I could forget it" (Burgess and Holmstrom 1979, p. 1280).

Nonetheless, complete avoidance of all reminders is unlikely to be successful, particularly when reminders may also include an individual's internal cognitions and feelings at the time of attempted suppression. Kuyken and Brewin (1994) found that women with a history of childhood sexual or physical abuse who were currently depressed reported both high levels of intrusive memories of the abuse and avoidance of those memories. This preliminary study did not permit the directionality of these effects to be determined (did intrusive memories lead to depression, or did depression encourage higher levels of intrusive memories?) nor did it include an assessment of the extent to which high intrusiveness and avoidance were especially true for memories of abuse as opposed to negative and stressful life events more generally. However, both the increased availability of negative thoughts and the decreased capacity for cognitive effort caused by depression could act to undermine attempts at suppression (see, for example, Conway et al. 1991; see also Freeston et al. 1995) by enhancing similarity to the original context in which suppression had occurred and by diminishing the ability to find or devise effective distractor thoughts.

The Interconnectedness of Intentional Forgetting and Thought Suppression With Other Factors That May Affect Memory

A self-initiated effort to avoid thoughts or memories of abuse may interact with and supplement factors in the environment that encourage thought suppression and forgetting. The press toward secrecy or discomfort experienced when discussing an incident may decrease the extent to which thoughts about the incident are elaborated and conceptualized (see Goodman et al. 1994; see also Fivush and Schwarzmueller 1995). Both self-initiated and externally encouraged efforts to suppress thoughts may either diminish or increase the formation of interassociations between thoughts about the abuse and other aspects of the individual's internal and external environment (e.g., Nelson 1993; Tessler and Nelson 1994). Although the latter possibility—that attempts at suppression will *increase* associative ties between the thought and the environment—is highlighted by the association hypothesis, the degree to which such interassociations are formed is also clearly moderated by the presence or absence of focused distractor techniques. For example, one account of the findings from Wegner and Gold (1995) that were discussed earlier in this chapter, in which only participants who had suppressed thoughts about a "cold flame" showed a rebound effect, focuses on the importance of environmental cuing together with distractors. Kelly and Kahn (1994) proposed that individuals thinking about a "cold flame" may not have been recently suppressing thoughts about him or her, so they were not prepared with salient or focused distractors. They may, therefore, have been more likely to use cues in the external laboratory environment to provide distraction, thereby also increasing the likelihood of later rebound due to environmental cuing.

Evidence indicates that individuals who have been abused may have fewer specific memories from childhood and may more often produce "overgeneral" autobiographical memories in response to word cues (see Kuyken and Brewin 1995; Parks and Balon 1995). These autobiographical memory deficits may partially result from diminished encoding or later elaboration and thinking of the times when abuse occurred (see J. M. G. Williams 1992). It is at least possible that poor memory for entire periods may reflect earlier efforts not to think of specific episodes by *also* not thinking of events, people, or places associated with abuse.

Likewise, cognitive changes due to development are not neatly separable from thought suppression or intentional forgetting. Although cognitive developmental changes may directly result in diminished memory caused by infantile or childhood amnesia (e.g., Howe et al. 1994; but cf. Nelson 1993), developmental factors may also affect the likelihood that intentional efforts at controlling memory will be undertaken and the probable success of such attempts. Discussing the interview responses of women with documented incidents of childhood abuse, L. M. Williams (1995) noted that some women reported that they did not immediately begin intentionally blocking out memories of the abuse but began doing so only some time later. On the one hand, as L. M. Williams (1995, p. 668) observed, this may be because developmental factors precluded the use of such strategies: "[D]eliberate forgetting may be available as a strategy only for the child who has attained more formal cognitive operations and has at least some limited verbal skills." On the other hand, as L. M. Williams also noted, because these reports were based on participants' subjective reports, documenting whether such *delayed* attempts at voluntary forgetting do, in fact, occur requires longitudinal research. More generally, the issue of the frequency of delayed attempts to forget trauma is important, especially because such delays may be more likely to be accompanied by aid from the environment in the form of contextual change and thus are more likely to be successful.

Self-reports including phrases such as "I blocked it out" or "I didn't think about it" do not convey how this occurs. Although, as observed at the outset, there is little reason to believe that there is a form of massive unconscious repression of traumatic incidents, the exact manner in which individuals use conscious efforts to not think about traumatic events is unclear. Does "blocking it out" involve a simple effort not to think about the event or the use of specific distractor thoughts? If so, how is distraction related to dissociation or to related factors such as imaginative involvement or absorption (e.g., Kihlstrom et al. 1994; Spiegel and Cardeña 1991; Tellegen and Atkinson 1974; see also Trickett and Putnam 1993)? Evidence from both the directed forgetting and thought suppression literature clearly shows that the use of focused distractors results in a more effective limitation of memory and thoughts than does unfocused distraction. How, more precisely, did individuals such as those cited earlier from the L. M. Williams study "block out" memories or thoughts of the abuse?

Finally, there is also a complex interplay of denial or blocking of *cognitive* information and the repression of *emotion* (e.g., Davis 1990; Weinberger et al. 1979). What role might the denial of the emotional effect of traumatic or stressful events, the isolation of affect, or affective blunting play in thought suppression or intentional forgetting? For example, in a recent case reported by Mann and Delon (1995, p. 503), a woman who had been raped at age 14 by her sister's fiancé confided that: "in previous years, memories of the rape had occasionally invaded her thoughts, but were infrequent and were associated with little affect." To what extent did emotional numbing render recall less likely to begin with? And—even if memories did invade her thoughts—to what extent did the emotional numbing preclude or curtail any cognitive processing and elaboration of those memories, thereby also rendering future retrievals less likely? Although some evidence indicates that successful cognitive suppression may not necessarily be accompanied by successful emotional suppression (Wegner et al. 1990), it is also probable that cognitive suppression may at times "benefit" from emotional suppression (see, for example, Holtgraves and Hall 1995; Kuhl 1985; Tomarken and Davidson 1994).

Future Directions and Questions

Research on voluntary thought suppression has been limited in that it has primarily examined factors that influence the frequency of the to-be-suppressed target thought on a short-term basis and following a *counterinstruction* that explicitly encourages or implicitly permits the occurrence of the target thought. However, this research cannot inform us as to what would happen if individuals persisted unabated in a continued attempt to suppress the target thought. To be effective, perhaps suppression does not need to be absolutely or entirely successful directly from the beginning. Initial expression or thinking about an episode followed by thought suppression ultimately might be a more effective way to forget. Research exploring the consequences of a more sustained long-term effort to suppress, particularly after different degrees of initial elaboration and expression of the thought, is especially needed.

Likewise, as noted earlier in this chapter, further research on contextual factors in directed forgetting, particularly when larger episodes are involved (block cuing), is also needed. Research employing multidimensional and complex materials, especially emotionally significant materials, would be particularly valuable. In addition, it would be informative to begin to explore item cuing and block cuing within individuals rather than only across individuals. If the processes involved in the two procedures are, indeed, fundamentally different, are individuals especially adept at one form and not the other? Can individuals become more proficient at forgetting with appropriate instructions? The results of the study by Geiselman et al. (1985), discussed earlier, in which subjects who were instructed to use the mental "STOP" procedure rather than other less active and less focused strategies showed greater forgetting, suggest that more explicit strategy instructions may well enhance forgetting. However, comparable studies using the block-cuing procedure would also be informative. Also, many studies would benefit from a focus not only on the consequences of suppression or attempted forgetting on recall or recognition of the to-be-forgotten information but also on the degree to which memory for the target episodes corresponds to the earlier events—memory accuracy as well as accessibility (see Koriat and Goldsmith 1996). Explorations of the accessibility of contextual information under directed forgetting with the block-cuing procedure suggest that errors in monitoring the source of information (e.g., M. K. Johnson et al. 1993) might be especially pronounced for material that was earlier subjected to the intention to forget. What are the hazards for memory accuracy arising from attempts to consciously forget? Are the impairments in source memory documented thus far with the block-cuing method (Geiselman et al. 1983; Koutstaal 1996) due to the involvement of contextual representations in initiating forgetting in the first place? Or might more general decrements in accuracy be observed?

Horowitz (1986, cited in Greenberg 1995, p. 1283) has differentiated three types of adaptive control that a traumatized individual might exercise over intrusive cognitions: "(a) control over when, where, in what manner, and for how long the trauma is contemplated; (b) control over the self-concepts and world views that guide the review; and (c) control over what information about the trauma is considered and what is disregarded." Neither obsessive rumination nor complete failure to cognitively and emotionally work through trauma is likely to result in optimal adjustment. Nonetheless, a certain degree of intentional forgetting may in some—possibly many—cases ultimately prove to be a healthy response. An intrusive and too pervasive concern with abuse may undermine what one hopes to establish: present and future relationships that move beyond exploitation, toward increasing strength and autonomy. On the one hand, insufficient conscious awareness and emotional and conceptual understanding of the nature and ramifications of the abuse may leave individuals vulnerable to harmful consequences of abuse, including the possibility of repeated abuse. On the other hand, excessive intrusiveness of the abuse into consciousness and preoccupation with the abusive episodes also may leave individuals vulnerable and diminish functioning at all levels. Seeking greater understanding of when it is best to remember and when it is best to suppress or to forget is to some degree not only an open empirical question at the nomothetic level but also a deep empirical question—in the sense of rooted in experience—at the idiographic level. Nonetheless, experimental research can also provide guidance at this level and may ultimately provide understanding not only of the conditions that may allow survival but also of successful overcoming and healing.

References

Adams-Tucker C: Proximate effects of sexual abuse in children: a report on 28 children. Am J Psychiatry 139:1252–1256, 1982

Allen JJ, Iacono WG, Laravuso JJ, et al: An event-related potential investigation of post-hypnotic recognition amnesia. J Abnorm Psychol 104:421–430, 1995

Barnhardt TM: Directed forgetting effects in explicit and implicit memory. Ph.D. Dissertation, University of Arizona, 1993

Basden BH, Basden DR: Directed forgetting: further comparisons of the item and list methods. Memory (in press)

Basden BH, Basden DR, Gargano GJ: Directed forgetting in implicit and explicit memory tests: a comparison of methods. J Exp Psychol Learn Mem Cogn 19:603–616, 1993a

Basden BH, Basden DR, Torzynski R: Directed forgetting in conceptual and perceptual implicit tests. Paper presented at the meeting of the Psychonomics Society, St. Louis, MO, November 1993b

Basden BH, Basden DR, Coe WC, et al: Retrieval inhibition in directed forgetting and posthypnotic amnesia. Int J Clin Exp Hypn 42:184–203, 1994

Beckmann J: Ruminative thought and the deactivation of an intention. Motivation and Emotion 18:317–334, 1994

Bjork RA: Retrieval inhibition as an adaptive mechanism in human memory, in Varieties of Memory and Consciousness: Essays in Honour of Endel Tulving. Edited by Roediger HL III, Craik FIM. Hillsdale, NJ, Lawrence Erlbaum, 1989, pp 309–330

Bjork RA, Bjork EL: Dissociations in the impact of to-be-forgotten information on memory. Paper presented at the annual meeting of the American Psychological Association, San Francisco, CA, August 1991

Bjork RA, Geiselman RE: Constituent processes in the differentiation of items in memory. J Exp Psychol Hum Learn Mem 4:347–361, 1978

Brandt J, Rubinsky E, Lassen G: Uncovering malingered amnesia. Ann N Y Acad Sci 444:502–503, 1985

Bray NW, Justice EM, Zahm DN: Two developmental transitions in selective remembering strategies. J Exp Child Psychol 36:43–55, 1983

Bray NW, Hersh RE, Turner LA: Selective remembering during adolescence. Developmental Psychology 21:290–294, 1985

Browne A, Finkelhor D: Impact of child sexual abuse: a review of the research. Psychol Bull 99:66–77, 1986

Burgess AW, Holmstrom LL: Adaptive strategies and recovery from rape. Am J Psychiatry 136:1278–1282, 1979

Christenson RM, Walker JM, Ross DR, et al: Reactivation of traumatic conflicts. Am J Psychiatry 138:984–985, 1981

Clark DM, Ball S, Pape D: An experimental investigation of thought suppression. Behav Res Ther 29:253–257, 1991

Clark DM, Winton E, Thynn L: A further experimental investigation of thought suppression. Behav Res Ther 31:207–210, 1993

Conte JR, Wolf S, Smith T: What sexual offenders tell us about prevention strategies. Child Abuse Negl 13:293–301, 1989

Conway M, Howell A, Giannopoulos C: Dysphoria and thought suppression. Cognitive Therapy and Research 15:153–166, 1991

Craik FIM, Tulving E: Depth of processing and the retention of words in episodic memory. J Exp Psychol Gen 104:268–294, 1975

Crowne DP, Marlowe D: The Approval Motive: Studies in Evaluative Dependence. New York, Wiley, 1964

Davies G, Thomson DM (eds): Memory in Context: Context in Memory. Chichester, Sussex, England, Wiley, 1988

Davis PJ: Repression and the inaccessibility of emotional memories, in Repression and Dissociation: Implications for Personality Theory, Psychopathology, and Health. Edited by Singer JL. Chicago, IL, University of Chicago Press, 1990, pp 387–403

Eisen MR: Return of the repressed: hypnoanalysis of a case of total amnesia. Int J Clin Exp Hypn 37:107–119, 1989

Epstein W, Wilder L: Searching for to-be-forgotten material in a directed forgetting task. J Exp Psychol 95:349–357, 1972

Everson MD, Hunter WM, Runyan DK, et al: Maternal support following disclosure of incest. Am J Orthopsychiatry 59:197–207, 1989

Feldman-Summers S, Pope KS: The experience of "forgetting" childhood abuse: a national survey of psychologists. J Consult Clin Psychol 62:636–639, 1994

Finkelhor D, Hotaling G, Lewis IA, et al: Sexual abuse in a national survey of adult men and women. Child Abuse Negl 14:19–28, 1990

Fivush R, Schwarzmueller A: Say it once again: effects of repeated questions on children's event recall. J Trauma Stress 8:555–580, 1995

Freeston MH, Ladouceur R, Provencher M, et al: Strategies used with intrusive thoughts: context, appraisal, mood, and efficacy. Journal of Anxiety Disorders 9:201–215, 1995

Gardiner JM, Java R: Recognition memory and awareness: an experiential approach. European Journal of Cognitive Psychology 5:337–346, 1993

Gardiner JM, Gawlik B, Richardson-Klavehn A: Maintenance rehearsal affects knowing not remembering; elaborative rehearsal affects remembering, not knowing. Psychonomic Bulletin and Review 1:107–110, 1994

Geiselman RE, Panting TM: Personality correlates of retrieval processes in intentional and unintentional forgetting. Personality and Individual Differences 6:685–691, 1985

Geiselman RE, Bjork RA, Fishman DL: Disrupted retrieval in directed forgetting: a link with posthypnotic amnesia. J Exp Psychol Gen 112:58–72, 1983

Geiselman RE, Rabow VE, Wachtel SL, et al: Strategy control in intentional forgetting. Human Learning 4:169–178, 1985

Goernert PN, Larson ME: The initiation and release of retrieval inhibition. J Gen Psychol 12:61–66, 1994

Golding JM, Long DL, MacLeod CM: You can't always forget what you want: directed forgetting of related words. Journal of Memory and Language 33:493–510, 1994

Goodman GS, Quas JA, Batterman-Faunce JM, et al: Predictors of accurate and inaccurate memories of traumatic events experienced in childhood. Consciousness and Cognition 3:269–294, 1994

Goschke T, Kuhl J: Representation of intentions: persisting activation in memory. J Exp Psychol Learn Mem Cogn 19:1211–1227, 1993

Greenberg MA: Cognitive processing of traumas: the role of intrusive thoughts and reappraisals. Journal of Applied Social Psychology 25:1262–1296, 1995

Harnishfeger KK, Pope RS: Intending to forget: the development of cognitive inhibition in directed forgetting. J Exp Child Psychol 62:292–315, 1996

Hasher L, Zacks RT: Automatic and effortful processes in memory. J Exp Psychol Gen 108:356–388, 1979

Holmes DS: The evidence for repression: an examination of sixty years of research, in Repression and Dissociation: Implications for Personality Theory, Psychopathology, and Health. Edited by Singer JL. Chicago, IL, University of Chicago Press, 1990, pp 85–102

Holtgraves T, Hall R: Repressors: what do they repress and how do they repress it? Journal of Research in Personality 29:306–317, 1995

Homa D, Spieker S: Assessment of selective search as an explanation for intentional forgetting. J Exp Psychol 103:10–15, 1974

Horowitz MJ: Stress Response Syndromes, 2nd Edition. Northvale, NJ, Jason Aronson, 1986

Howard DV: Search and decision processes in intentional forgetting: a reaction time analysis. J Exp Psychol Hum Learn Mem 2:566–576, 1976

Howard DV, Goldin SE: Selective processing in encoding and memory: an analysis of resource allocation by kindergarten children. J Exp Child Psychol 27:87–95, 1979

Howe ML, Courage ML, Peterson C: How can I remember when "I" wasn't there: long-term retention of traumatic experiences and emergence of the cognitive self. Consciousness and Cognition 3:327–355, 1994

Howell A, Conway M: Mood and the suppression of positive and negative self-referent thoughts. Cognitive Therapy and Research 16:535–555, 1992

Johnson HM: Processes of successful intentional forgetting. Psychol Bull 116:274–292, 1994

Johnson MK, Hashtroudi S, Lindsay DS: Source monitoring. Psychol Bull 114:3–28, 1993

Kanak NJ, Stevens R: PI and RI in serial learning as a function of environmental context. Applied Cognitive Psychology 6:589–606, 1992

Kelly AE, Kahn JH: Effects of suppression of personal intrusive thoughts. J Pers Soc Psychol 66:998–1006, 1994

Kihlstrom JF, Glisky MI, Anguilo MJ: Dissociative tendencies and dissociative disorders. J Abnorm Psychol 103:117–124, 1994

Koriat A, Goldsmith M: Memory metaphors and the real-life/laboratory controversy: correspondence versus storehouse conceptions of memory. Behavioral Brain Science 19:167–228, 1996

Koutstaal W: Beyond content: The fate—or function?—of contextual information in directed forgetting. Ph.D. Dissertation, Harvard University, 1996

Koutstaal W, Schacter DL: Inaccuracy and inaccessibility in memory retrieval: contributions from cognitive psychology and neuropsychology, in Trauma and Memory: Clinical and Legal Controversies. Edited by Appelbaum PS, Uyehara LA, Elin MR. New York, Oxford University Press (in press)

Krystal JH, Bennet AL, Bremner JD, et al: Toward a cognitive neuroscience of dissociation and altered memory functions in post-traumatic stress disorder, in Neurobiological and Clinical Consequences of Stress: From Normal Adaptation to PTSD. Edited by Friedman MJ, Charney DS, Deutch AY. Philadelphia, PA, Lippincott-Raven, 1995, pp 239–269

Kuhl J: Volitional mediators of cognition-behavior consistency: self-regulatory processes and action versus state orientation, in Action Control: From Cognition to Behavior. Edited by Kuhl J, Beckmann J. New York, Springer-Verlag, 1985, pp 101–128

Kumar K, Wilkinson JCM: Thought stopping: a useful treatment in phobias of 'internal stimuli.' Br J Psychiatry 119:305–307, 1971

Kuyken W, Brewin CR: Intrusive memories of childhood abuse during depressive episodes. Behav Res Ther 32:525–528, 1994

Kuyken W, Brewin CR: Autobiographical memory functioning in depression and reports of early abuse. J Abnorm Psychol 104:585–591, 1995

Lane JD, Wegner DM: The cognitive consequences of secrecy. J Pers Soc Psychol 69:237–253, 1995

Lavy EH, van den Hout MA: Cognitive avoidance and attentional bias: causal relationships. Cognitive Therapy and Research 18:179–191, 1994

Lockhart RS: Conceptual specificity in thinking and remembering, in Memory in Context: Context in Memory. Edited by Davies GM, Thomson DM. Chichester, Sussex, England, Wiley, 1988, pp 319–331

Loftus E: The reality of repressed memories. Am Psychol 48:518–537, 1993

MacLeod C: Directed forgetting affects both direct and indirect tests of memory. J Exp Psychol Learn Mem Cogn 15:13–21, 1989

Macrae CN, Bodenhausen GV, Milne AB, et al: Out of mind but back in sight: stereotypes on the rebound. J Pers Soc Psychol 67:808–817, 1994

Mann SJ, Delon M: Improved hypertension control after disclosure of decades-old trauma. Psychosom Med 57:501–505, 1995

Mathews A, Milroy R: Effects of priming and suppression of worry. Behav Res Ther 32:843–850, 1994

McGee R: Flashbacks and memory phenomena: a comment on "flashback phenomena—clinical and diagnostic dilemmas." J Nerv Ment Dis 172:273–278, 1984

McGeoch JA: Forgetting and the law of disuse. Psychol Rev 39:352–370, 1932

Muris P, Merckelbach H, van den Hout M, et al: Suppression of emotional and neutral material. Behav Res Ther 30:639–642, 1992

Muris P, Merckelbach H, de Jong P: Verbalization and environmental cuing in thought suppression. Behav Res Ther 31:609–612, 1993

Myers LB, Brewin CR, Power MJ: Repression and autobiographical memory, in Theoretical Perspectives on Autobiographical Memory. Edited by Conway MA, Rubin DC, Spinnler H, et al. Dordrecht, The Netherlands, Kluwer Academic, 1992, pp 375–390

Nader K, Pynoos R, Fairbanks L, et al: Children's PTSD reactions one year after a sniper attack at their school. Am J Psychiatry 147:1526–1530, 1990

Nash MR: Memory distortion and sexual trauma: the problem of false negatives and false positives. Int J Clin Exp Hypn 42:346–362, 1994

Nelson K: The psychological and social origins of autobiographical memory. Psychological Science 4:1–8, 1993

Ofshe RJ, Singer MT: Recovered-memory therapy and robust repression: influence and pseudomemories. Int J Clin Exp Hypn 42:391–410, 1994

Parks ED, Balon R: Autobiographical memory for childhood events: patterns of recall in psychiatric patients with a history of alleged trauma. Psychiatry 58:199–208, 1995

Pope HG Jr, Hudson JI: Can memories of childhood sexual abuse be "repressed"? Psychol Med 25:121–126, 1995

Putnam FW: Dissociative disorders in children: behavioral profiles and problems. Child Abuse Negl 17:39–45, 1993

Roediger HL III, Crowder RC: Instructed forgetting: rehearsal control or retrieval inhibition (repression)? Cognitive Psychology 3:244–254, 1972

Roediger HL III, Weldon MS, Challis BH: Explaining dissociations between implicit and explicit measures of retention: a processing account, in Varieties of Memory and Consciousness: Essays in Honour of Endel Tulving. Edited by Roediger HL, Craik FIM. Hillsdale, NJ, Lawrence Erlbaum, 1989, pp 3–41

Roemer L, Borkovec TD: Effects of suppressing thoughts about emotional material. J Abnorm Psychol 103:467–474, 1994

Salkovskis PM, Campbell P: Thought suppression induces intrusion in naturally occurring negative intrusive thoughts. Behav Res Ther 32:1–8, 1994

Schacter DL: Feeling-of-knowing ratings distinguish between genuine and simulated forgetting. J Exp Psychol Learn Mem Cogn 12:30–41, 1986

Schacter DL: Priming and multiple memory systems: perceptual mechanisms of implicit memory, in Memory Systems 1994. Edited by Schacter DL, Tulving E. Cambridge, MA, MIT Press, 1994, pp 233–268

Schacter DL: Searching for Memory: The Brain, the Mind, and the Past. New York, Basic Books, 1996

Schacter DL, Wang PL, Tulving E, et al: Functional retrograde amnesia: a quantitative case study. Neuropsychologia 20:523–532, 1982

Schacter DL, Kihlstrom JF, Kihlstrom LC, et al: Autobiographical memory in a case of multiple personality disorder. J Abnorm Psychol 98:508–514, 1989

Schacter DL, Norman KA, Koutstaal W: The recovered memory debate: a cognitive neuroscience perspective, in False and Recovered Memories. Edited by Conway MA. New York, Oxford University Press (in press)

Schooler JW: Seeking the core: the issues and evidence surrounding recovered accounts of sexual trauma. Consciousness and Cognition 3:452–469, 1994

Silver RL, Boon C, Stones MH: Searching for meaning in misfortune: making sense of incest. Journal of Social Issues 39:81–102, 1983

Smith SM: Mood is a component of mental context: comment on Eich (1995). J Exp Psychol Gen 124:309–310, 1995

Spanos NP, James B, DeGroot HP: Detection of simulated hypnotic amnesia. J Abnorm Psychol 99:179–182, 1990

Spiegel D: Hypnosis and suggestion, in Memory Distortion: How Minds, Brains, and Societies Reconstruct the Past. Edited by Schacter DL, Coyle JT, Fischbach GD, et al. Cambridge, MA, Harvard University Press, 1995, pp 129–149

Spiegel D, Cardeña E: Disintegrated experience: the dissociative disorders revisited. J Abnorm Psychol 100:366–378, 1991

Taylor J: A personality scale of manifest anxiety. J Abnorm Soc Psychol 48:285–290, 1953

Tellegen A, Atkinson G: Openness to absorbing and self-altering experiences ("absorption"), a trait related to hypnotic susceptibility. J Abnorm Psychol 83:268–277, 1974

Tessler M, Nelson K: Making memories: the influence of joint encoding on later recall by young children. Consciousness and Cognition 3:307–326, 1994

Tomarken AJ, Davidson RJ: Frontal brain activation in repressors and nonrepressors. J Abnorm Psychol 103:339–349, 1994

Trickett PK, Putnam FW: Impact of child sexual abuse on females: toward a developmental, psychobiological integration. Psychological Science 4:81–87, 1993

Trinder H, Salkovskis PM: Personally relevant intrusions outside the laboratory: long-term suppression increases intrusion. Behav Res Ther 32:833–842, 1994

Tulving E: Elements of Episodic Memory. Oxford, UK, Clarendon Press, 1983

Tulving E, Pearlstone Z: Availability versus accessibility of information in memory for words. Journal of Verbal Learning and Verbal Behavior 5:381–391, 1966

Turner SM, Holzman A, Jacob RG: Treatment of compulsive looking by imaginal thought-stopping. Behav Modif 7:576–582, 1983

Uleman JS: A framework for thinking intentionally about unintended thoughts, in Unintended Thought. Edited by Uleman JS, Bargh JA. New York, Guilford, 1989, pp 425–449

Wegner DM: White Bears and Other Unwanted Thoughts. New York, Guilford, 1994

Wegner DM, Erber R: The hyperaccessibility of suppressed thoughts. J Pers Soc Psychol 63:903–912, 1992

Wegner DM, Gold DB: Fanning old flames: emotional and cognitive effects of suppressing thoughts of a past relationship. J Pers Soc Psychol 68:782–792, 1995

Wegner DM, Schneider DJ, Carter SR III, et al: Paradoxical effects of thought suppression. J Pers Soc Psychol 53:5–13, 1987

Wegner DM, Shortt JW, Blake AW, et al: The suppression of exciting thoughts. J Pers Soc Psychol 58:409–418, 1990

Wegner DM, Schneider DJ, Knutson B, et al: Polluting the stream of consciousness: the effect of thought suppression on the mind's environment. Cognitive Therapy and Research 15:141–152, 1991

Wegner DM, Erber R, Zanakos S: Ironic processes in the mental control of mood and mood-related thought. J Pers Soc Psychol 65:1093–1104, 1993

Weinberger DA, Schwartz GE, Davidson RJ: Low-anxious, high-anxious, and repressive coping styles: psychometric patterns and behavioral and physiological responses to stress. J Abnorm Psychol 88:369–380, 1979

Weiner B: Motivated forgetting and the study of repression. J Pers 36:213–234, 1968

Wenzlaff RM, Wegner DM, Roper DW: Depression and mental control: the resurgence of unwanted negative thoughts. J Pers Soc Psychol 55:882–892, 1988

Wenzlaff RM, Wegner DM, Klein SB: The role of thought suppression in the bonding of thought and mood. J Pers Soc Psychol 60:500–508, 1991

Williams JMG: Autobiographical memory and emotional disorders, in The Handbook of Emotion and Memory: Research and Theory. Edited by Christianson S-A. Hillsdale, NJ, Lawrence Erlbaum, 1992, pp 451–477

Williams LM: Recall of childhood trauma: a prospective study of women's memories of child sexual abuse. J Consult Clin Psychol 62:1167–1176, 1994

Williams LM: Recovered memories of abuse in women with documented child sexual victimization histories. J Trauma Stress 8:649–673, 1995

Williamsen JA, Johnson HJ, Eriksen CW: Some characteristics of posthypnotic amnesia. J Abnorm Psychol 70:123–131, 1965

Chapter 9

Perspectives on Adult Memories of Childhood Sexual Abuse: A Research Review

Linda M. Williams, Ph.D., and Victoria L. Banyard, Ph.D.

Adult memories and recollection of childhood sexual abuse are the focus of both increasing interest and continuing controversy for researchers, clinicians, and lawyers in the field of child maltreatment. News of cases of recovered memories for sexual abuse and opposing views about the veracity of such accounts have appeared in media ranging from the popular press to academic journals and conference symposia. No longer is the focus of media attention on the incidence and prevalence of child sexual abuse, drawing attention to the seriousness of a long hidden problem. Indeed, a recent review of the coverage of the issue of child sexual abuse in the popular news media found that 73% of the articles about child sexual abuse during 1992–1994 were focused on the issue of false accusations in general. In 1994, 65% of the articles on child sexual abuse dealt with the specific issue of false memories (Beckett 1996), portraying recovered memories of abuse as unreliable and emphasizing the damage false accusations do to families and wrongly accused individuals. Beckett suggests that this refocus of public attention on false allegations may be a consequence of increased attention to cases of abuse in which family members were the perpetrators. When abuse is seen as a threat to children by dangerous "outsiders," then the societal response is unified or solidaristic. However, when alleged perpetrators are insiders such as family members (Beckett 1996), or community leaders such as priests, judges, and other professionals, the social fabric is disrupted and a social denial is elicited.

Achieving a better understanding of memory for traumatic events is crucial for both researchers who study the effects of child maltreatment and clinicians who work with trauma survivors. Andrews et al. (1995) surveyed British psychotherapists and found that 51% of therapists who worked with sexually abused patients reported that they had seen patients who, during some period, did not have a clear memory for the sexual abuse. Proponents of different sides of this debate have

This research was supported by the U.S. Department of Health and Human Services, National Center on Child Abuse and Neglect, Grant 90-CA-1552.

cautioned practitioners against what they see as the widespread use of *memory recovery therapy,* the danger of creating false memories in the minds of those in treatment for emotional problems (Lindsay and Read 1994), and the negative consequences of being unsupportive of memory recovery (Herman 1992). Clearly, the questions about memory and child sexual abuse are important for anyone practicing in the field of child maltreatment. To understand this issue, however, it is necessary to look beyond the rhetoric and to examine what we really know about this phenomenon. Such is the aim of this chapter. We review and synthesize recent empirical findings on the impact of childhood sexual abuse on adult memory by drawing from a diverse empirical literature from the fields of cognitive, developmental, and clinical psychology; psychiatry; and child maltreatment.

We consider several basic questions in this chapter:

1. Are memories of childhood events different from memories of adulthood experiences because of developmental differences in the structure of memory systems of children and adults?
2. Is memory for trauma different, or does it operate in different ways, from everyday, declarative memory?
3. Do memories of childhood sexual abuse at any age differ qualitatively from memories of other events, even memories of other trauma?

We must ask not only how the experience of trauma may influence memory but also how the experience of sexual abuse may influence memory. In the second section of this chapter, we consider the empirical evidence that supports the likelihood that childhood sexual abuse can be forgotten, that memories of childhood sexual abuse can be implanted, and that memories of such abuse, once forgotten, can be recovered.

A Developmental Perspective on Memory

An extensive body of research on adult memory and memory for autobiographical events has raised a number of important issues. Research on memory processes more generally, for example, has shown that memory is imperfect (Rogers 1995), although investigators disagree about the degree to which memory is fallible and under what conditions (Brewin et al. 1993; Henry et al. 1994). Various studies suggest that all experiences or aspects of experiences are not encoded and stored and that more experience is in fact forgotten than is remembered (Lindsay and Read 1994; Squire 1989). Other work has focused on the conditions under which memory errors occur. Research has shown that the memory of both adults and children may be affected by the way that questions are asked, the presentation of new or misleading information, or prior knowledge (Belli and Loftus 1994; Ceci et al. 1981; Hyman and Pentland 1996; Loftus and Davies 1984; Loftus et al. 1992).

In addition to the general comment that memory is fallible, to understand memory function more fully requires taking a developmental perspective. This is particularly true if we wish to understand the process of memory as it pertains to sexual abuse experienced in childhood. Many different theories exist about the development of the memory system in childhood and about when memories are possible and how accurate they are (see Howe and Courage 1993 or Pillemer and White 1989 for extensive reviews of this literature).

Of particular interest to developmentalists and memory researchers has been the observation that adults do not seem to have any memories of events that occurred earlier than age 2–4 years. This phenomenon has been called "infantile" or "childhood amnesia" (Nelson 1988) and has been the subject of much theoretical discussion. Some researchers have posited that memory operates differently in childhood and in adulthood and that this explains the lack of adult memories for early childhood events. Nadel and Zola-Morgan (1984), for example, stated that structural, neurological differences between memory systems available to infants and those available to older children/adults create this absence of early memories. Others assert that the main differences are cognitive in nature (Usher and Neisser 1993), suggesting that childhood memories are encoded differently from adult memories or that lack of verbal skills in young children makes retrieval of information from that time impossible (Nelson and Ross 1980). Pillemer and White (1989) have even posited the existence of two independent memory systems—one that operates from birth and can process very general memories for various skills and routines and a second that develops later in early childhood that enables the individual to retain memories for more specific events and information. In a recent article, Schacter et al. (1995) review research that draws some limited parallels between memory errors made by children and those of patients with damage to the frontal lobe. Although Schacter and colleagues raised more questions than they answered, their review suggested a hypothesis that developmental differences in frontal-lobe maturity may partially account for age differences in memory errors, and they urge more research to be conducted in this area. What all these researchers have in common is the shared hypothesis that the memory systems of infants and young children have some type of structural differences that interfere with the long-term retention or accessibility of memories of events that occurred during this time.

In contrast, another group of researchers dispute the notion of a phenomenon such as infantile amnesia. They assert that no empirical evidence indicates differences in the memory systems of young children and adults. Memory, according to this view, does not become reorganized at some point in childhood but remains the same for children as it is for adults (Fivush and Hammond 1990; Howe and Courage 1993; Nelson 1988). They explain adults' lack of early memories by examining other aspects of cognitive and social development that affect the memory system. Fivush and Reese (1992), for example, discuss the fact that children seem to learn social rules for what is important to remember through conversations with parents. The lack of these rules early in childhood may lead to memories that are fragmented and difficult to retrieve and the appearance of infantile amnesia. Howe and Courage (1993) pay particular attention to the cognitive development of the child's sense of self. They assert that children have all the required memory systems at birth, but it is not until around age 2 years, when a coherent sense of self has developed, that true autobiographical memories about the self are possible. These theorists suggest that children's memory is not structurally any different from that of adults and that forgetting of childhood events may be related to other aspects of social and cognitive development more than to any developmental immaturity of the child's memory systems. Even these theories, however, raise questions about whether children can be expected to retain complex memories for events that occur before age 4 years.

Indeed, Goodman and colleagues' (1994) review of the literature on children's memories seems to show that regardless of whether memory structures are the same or different from that of adults, a variety of evidence indicates that some long-term retention of childhood events, particularly those that occur after age 4, as well as inaccessibility of these memories, is possible. Goodman et al. (1994) cited evidence that memories of young children, even after the period of disputed "infantile amnesia," may be more open to distortion by outside influences, and these young children may need more cues from others or the environment to recall certain events or information. Some aspects of memory develop over the course of childhood as children become more skilled at processes such as attaching meaning to memories. Such research suggests that, for developmental reasons, childhood events cannot always be expected to be clearly remembered. Goodman et al. (1994) also empirically examined children's memories of a traumatic and invasive medical procedure. Age predicted accurate recall of the event, and children age 5 years and older had more accurate memories that were less open to modification by outside information than did children ages 3 or 4. However, other, more individual, differences were also important—factors such as the emotional reaction of the child to the procedure (children who reported high levels of embarrassment had more memory errors), social support by a parent (children whose mothers were less supportive and talked with them less about the event had less accurate recall), and the child's prior knowledge of the medical procedure (children who had more knowledge had more accurate recall).

What are the implications of these studies of general memory processes for memories of traumatic events such as child sexual abuse? Again, this area of study is characterized by considerable controversy and disagreement. Some researchers suggest that memories for traumatic events are the same as for other events, suggesting that normal developmental differences in memories for childhood events may explain why some survivors of abuse have no or impaired recall of the trauma. Others provide evidence for a distinction, stating that trauma has unique effects on memory that may result in impaired recall. One avenue of investigation has examined the effect of emotion on memory based on the notion that the emotional salience of traumatic events may exert particular effects on memory.

The Impact of Emotion on Memory

Memory researchers have studied the impact of emotion on memory and have examined the question: "Are memories for highly emotionally salient events more clearly remembered?" Brown and Kulik (1977), for example, discussed their discovery of what they termed *flashbulb memories*. These are memories for highly salient and surprising events that seem to create permanent memories of even minute details of the situation, such as an imprint of the details of where one was at the time one learned of John F. Kennedy's assassination. Others, such as Rubin and Kozin (1984), have looked more broadly at "vivid memories," which seem to be associated with surprising and important events. Some have critiqued these theories and this research and asserted that memories such as "flashbulb memories" may not be accurate (Neisser, cited in Rubin and Kozin 1984). Although some research reports that high emotional arousal can lead to narrowing of one's attention and less accurate memories for details of the event or can decrease recall for other stimuli around or previous to the event (Burke et al. 1992; Kramer et al. 1991; Loftus and Burns 1982), in a review of this literature, Koss et al. (1995) found that "emotional memories have been characterized as 'detailed, accurate, and persistent' and ratings of intense emotional reaction are predictive of better, not worse, recall" (p. 124). In terms of sexual abuse, such theories would suggest that the central elements of traumatic events may be better remembered than those of nontraumatic events because of their emotional salience.

Memory for Traumatic Events Is the Same as That for Other Events

Overall, the evidence seems to indicate that central details of emotionally salient events are well remembered by individuals over time, but these memories are not immune to modifying influences (Howe et al. 1994; Loftus and Christianson 1989). However, are memories for traumatic events—situations in which emotional arousal is extremely high—different in some way from memories for more neutral events? A number of researchers do not believe so. Loftus and Christianson (1989), for example, did not find evidence that traumatic or highly emotional stimuli are more well remembered than other events and even suggested that they may be less well remembered than neutral stimuli and may be more susceptible to misinformation given after the memory has formed. Loftus (1993) asserted that evidence of forgetting incidents of childhood sexual abuse may be the result of the same process of forgetting that affects individuals' memories for any event and that no unique process is at work because the event is traumatic. Howe et al. (1994) conducted a study of children's memories of a traumatic injury that led to an emergency room visit. They concluded that these traumatic events were not remembered differently from other events. The degree of stress of the child was not related to how well the event was recalled. Furthermore, although central details of the event were reasonably well remembered even 6 months later, children's recollection of more peripheral details declined over time, as would be predicted by theories of normal forgetting. They stated:

> This finding is consistent with our proposal that traumatic and autobiographical events enjoy no special status in long-term memory. That is, unlike what some theorists would have us believe (e.g., Freud 1953), these memories are not held in some secret repository that is immune to the ravages of normal forgetting. Rather, like all memories, early autobiographical memories and memories for traumatic events are subject to the same laws that govern the retention of memories in general. (Howe et al. 1994, p. 347)

The points raised by such research are important to consider and highlight the ways in which memory systems may operate similarly across a variety of situations. There are some limitations, however. As Goodman et al. (1994) have discussed in relation to their own work on children's memories for hospitalizations, qualitative differences may persist between these emotionally difficult events and the types of trauma caused by child abuse or other life-threatening experiences such as rape and combat that may produce symptoms of posttraumatic stress disorder. These extreme forms of trauma may have a more direct and noticeable effect on memory systems.

Memory for Traumatic Events Is Different From That for Other Events

In contrast to the view that memories for traumatic events are the same as for any other experience, a number of researchers have discussed the ways in which traumatic memories may be different. These researchers tend to focus on the most extreme forms of traumatic events—child sexual abuse and wartime combat. Their research provides evidence that trauma does influence memory at the biological, psychological, and social levels. It creates the conditions for the formation of both indelible memories that continually reappear in consciousness through processes such as flashbacks and nightmares and pockets of amnesia for aspects of the traumatic experience.

van der Kolk has been one of the major proponents of this point of view (van der Kolk, in press; van der Kolk and Fisler 1995; van der Kolk and van der Hart 1991). van der Kolk has raised questions about whether the typical studies of trauma and memory that are conducted in the laboratory, where participants are shown a series of slides, some of which contain traumatic material such as watching a shooting, are really comparable to memory for real-life traumatic events. He and others assert that trauma can have profound physiological effects on brain structures such as the hippocampus that are key components of the memory system (see Bremner et al. 1995; Hartman and Burgess 1993; Siegel 1995; van der Kolk, in press, for a more extensive review of this literature). Prolonged stress responses that occur when an individual is traumatized may alter normal physiological stress and memory processes. This can lead to both "a strengthening of particular memory traces related to traumatic events, as well as gaps in memory, which are known as amnestic episodes" (Bremner et al. 1995, p. 531). This research is in its early stages but is further supported by studies such as that conducted by Cahill et al. (1994). They examined the hypothesis that better memory for emotionally salient events was related to activation of the β-adrenergic system. Human participants were divided into two groups—those who saw slides depicting a neutral story and those who saw a more emotional story about a boy in a life-threatening accident. Some participants were given a substance (propranolol) that blocks the β-adrenergic system, and others were given a placebo. The inhibitory substance had no effect on memory for the neutral stimulus but did decrease recall for details of the more emotionally salient event. This study demonstrates a link between the β-adrenergic system and memory and suggests ways in which physiological stress responses triggered by emotionally salient events can enhance memory for these events. These studies contribute to an understanding of how memories for traumatic events may be different and more indelible and well remembered.

In addition to differences in the physiology of traumatic events and memories of such events, recent research has also focused on psychological factors that may differentiate traumatic memories from others and thus explain why traumatic events may be less well remembered. van der Kolk and Fisler (1995), for example, presented some preliminary findings from a study of differences between traumatic and nontraumatic memories in patients with posttraumatic stress disorder. He found that the traumatic memories tended to be initially remembered "in the form of somatosensory or emotional flashback experiences" (p. 517). Traumatic memories seem to be experienced more in terms of bodily sensations, visual images, sounds, and so on rather than as a verbal narrative. van der Kolk used this finding as preliminary evidence to support his theory that memories of trauma may be initially sensorimotor in nature and may not be completely well organized. An individual may be, therefore, unable to verbalize the memory although she or he has some access to it. Enns et al. (1995) reviewed a variety of other research on cognitive theories of traumatic memory. They discussed the idea that trauma may affect cognitive information processing systems in several ways. It may lead to the use of dissociation or repression, mechanisms that limit information that is taken in or that can be retrieved from memory for the event. They also highlighted the ways in which trauma can disturb one's assumptions about oneself and one's world (Janoff-Bulman, cited in Enns et al. 1995). This threatening and inconsistent material may not easily fit into existing schemata about one's experience, and incomplete processing of this information may result (Enns et al. 1995).

Freyd (1994) also presented a theoretical argument for the effect of trauma on cognitive processing. She argued that amnesia may be an important survival strategy when an individual is confronted with traumatic stress, and sexual abuse in particular. As a coping strategy, "forgetting" one's abuse may allow one to maintain needed attachments to a perpetrator who may also be an important caregiver. She focused on the impact of traumatic betrayal as an important influence of trauma on memory. Although her discussion is purely theoretical, she concludes that "the degree to which a trauma involves a sense of having been fundamentally cheated or betrayed by another person may significantly influence the individual's cognitive encoding of the experience of trauma, the degree to which the event is easily accessible to awareness, and the psychological as well as behavioral responses" (p. 308).

Finally, the social context in which the trauma occurs and the ways in which social factors may affect the formation of traumatic memories have begun to be discussed. Fivush and Schwartzmuller (1995) reviewed research on how children recall events and the effect of questioning on children's reported memories. In this review, they suggested that a child's rehearsal of an event by talking to another person about it may aid the memory process. In situations in which the event is an incident of child abuse, however, this verbal rehearsing often may not occur because the event is kept secret. This may lead to impaired or less clear memories for such events. A study by Tromp et al. (1995) also speaks to the powerful role that silencing may play in the processing of traumatic memories for rape. They conducted a survey of 3,210 women, asking them to describe memories of a rape experience or other significant life event. They found that rape memories were different from other unpleasant memories in several important ways. Rape memories were rated as being more unpleasant and were also reported to be less well remembered and less talked and thought about. In their discussion of these results, the authors noted that victims of rape often remain silent about their experiences, and this silence may affect the memory process. Although research has not shown that events must be frequently talked or thought about in order to be remembered for any length of time, some investigators believe that sharing memories of events with others helps to change memories—to make them more connected to other memories and more integrated into one's experience. Tromp et al. (1995) hypothesized that when rape memories are not discussed, either because the victim cannot put her experiences into words or because she fears being blamed for the rape, these memories may not be erased but are simply kept outside of awareness and continue to influence her behavior or emotions because they have not been integrated into the larger scheme of her experience. van der Kolk and van der Hart (1991, p. 431) asserted that "in contrast to narrative memory, which is a social act, traumatic memory is inflexible and invariable. Traumatic memory has no social component; it is not addressed to anybody, the patient does not respond to anybody; it is a solitary activity."

Recall of Childhood Sexual Abuse

Thus far, the discussion of the research on memory has not permitted us to reach any definitive conclusions about memories of sexual abuse in childhood. Indeed, in many respects, more questions have been raised than answered. For example, Bremner and colleagues (1995) have found that child sexual abuse is associated with long-term deficits in verbal short-term memory. Their findings add to a growing literature that supports a relation between stress and alterations in memory. Neurobiological correlates of the effects of stress on memory may provide potential explanations for delayed recall of memories of childhood sexual abuse, but studies to date have provided only an incomplete picture of this phenomenon.

Much of the current controversy around this issue is fueled by contradictory research findings and a wide variety of difficulties encountered in conducting research on this topic (Carlson 1996). One of the difficulties in understanding the nature of adults' memories of childhood sexual abuse is that these are real, not laboratory-derived, events. The characteristics of the abuse and its timing cannot be controlled by researchers. It is also difficult to construct good analogue studies of memories of abuse, although some research with children has examined memories of interpersonal touching (Leippe et al. 1991) and medical procedures that involve the genitalia (Goodman et al. 1994; Saywitz et al. 1991). A complication of naturalistic studies of memory for sexual abuse is that child molestation usually occurs in private, and only rarely are other adults or even other children present. Thus, follow-up studies of memories of such abuse are plagued by incomplete data on what actually transpired during the abuse. Corroboration may simply be unavailable in most cases.

Research has documented the relevant characteristics of child sexual abuse (e.g., secrecy, threats of harm to child or others, grooming of the child to accept the sexual contact) that might dramatically affect memories of these events in ways that differ from memories of other types of traumatic childhood events (e.g., witnessing the death of a parent). Nevertheless, most of what is known about the dynamics and patterns of child sexual abuse comes from retrospective reports of adults molested during childhood (Finkelhor 1979; Herman 1992; Russell 1986) or perpetrators of the abuse (Conte et al. 1989; Williams and Finkelhor 1995) and is subject to possible distortion, confabulation, and other errors of memory.

Researchers have used a simple 2 × 2 table to examine the intersection of true abuse status (not abused/abused) and memory status (recalls/does not recall) (McHugh 1994; Spiegel 1993). Figure 9–1 is a

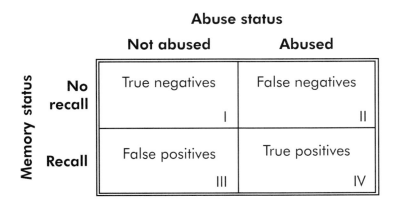

Figure 9–1. A 2 × 2 table of abuse and memory status.

diagram of this 2×2 table. Quadrant I represents those who were not abused and recall no abuse experiences (true negatives). Quadrant II includes those who were abused but do not recall the abuse (false negatives). Quadrant III represents those who were not abused but recall such experiences (false positives). Quadrant IV includes those who were abused and recall the abuse (true positives).

Consideration of the 2×2 table brings into focus a number of important issues in the debate about memories of childhood sexual abuse. The research and the theoretical focus of trauma researchers have centered on the right side of this table (false negatives and true positives), because these quadrants comprise all those who have been abused. The negative consequences of abuse and the symptomatology that brings many adult survivors of abuse in quadrant IV into contact with the medical and mental health systems have been well documented (Beitchman et al. 1992; Briere 1992; Browne and Finkelhor 1986). The work of trauma researchers has also focused on the problem of false negatives (quadrant II). At first, clinicians and researchers concentrated on false negatives attributable not to the victim's actual memory of the abuse but to the inadequacy of screening questions, for example, when a social and psychological history was taken on individuals presenting with psychiatric symptoms. It has been observed that asking behaviorally specific questions about abuse history or asking detailed questions about trauma history readily uncovers such histories in many patients (Briere and Zaidi 1989). Only relatively recently has attention been directed to the problems of truly forgotten abuse among clinical samples (Briere 1992; Courtois 1992; Herman 1992; L. Terr, "True memories of childhood trauma: quirks, absences, and returns," unpublished manuscript, Langley Porter Psychiatric Institute, University of California–San Francisco, 1994). Research in these areas has involved clinical, not laboratory, work.

On the other hand, researchers and practitioners concerned with the problem of false accusations have focused on the lower half of the 2×2 table, especially quadrant III (false positives). It is interesting that the label of "false memory" has come to be used to describe "false memories of abuse when such abuse did not really happen," but this label has not been used to refer to "false memories of no abuse when such abuse did indeed occur" (false negatives). In part, because the work of researchers in this area is driven by issues of criminal or civil defense (see Neimark 1996), significant attention has been given to examination of forensic issues, and laboratory research has attended to confabulation and errors of memory. Much of the work in this area has focused on suggestibility and problems of source attribution (i.e., the memory errors that arise when an individual recalls information that came from some source after the event and when that individual goes on to erroneously attribute the information to the original event).

Much of the debate about memory of childhood sexual abuse has focused on how cases are distributed among each of the quadrants in Figure 9–1 and on the explanations for how and why individuals come to falsely believe that they were not abused when, in fact, they were abused and to falsely believe that they were abused when, in fact, they were not. Some of the contentiousness (Berliner and Loftus 1992) in this false memory debate may have occurred because of communication errors, the differential attention paid to each quadrant by trauma researchers and memory researchers, different strategies for clinical and laboratory research, and the application of clinical research methods to quadrants II and IV and laboratory research designs to quadrant III. There has been little crossover in either direction to date. In the next several sections of this chapter, we review relevant research in the second, third, and fourth quadrants of the figure: false negatives, false positives, and true positives.

Forgetting Childhood Sexual Abuse—False Negatives

One critical research question at the root of the debate on "recovered" memory is, "How common is it to have no memory of sexual abuse that occurred in one's childhood?" People forget myriad ordinary experiences, but do people forget childhood sexual abuse, especially if the abuse was traumatic and occurred after the offset of infantile amnesia? This question has been raised repeatedly in the debate about memories of childhood sexual abuse. Loftus (1995) and others (Pope and Hudson 1995; Wakefield and Underwager 1991) have suggested that to have no recall of abuse is uncommon and argue that no evidence indicates that a child would forget a truly traumatic event unless the event occurred before age 3 years. However, other research documents the prevalence of this phenomenon.

Much of the research specifically focused on adults' experiences with forgetting childhood sexual abuse is based on naturalistic studies of clinical samples of women and men in treatment for the consequences of sexual abuse. This research reveals that many adults who recall sexual abuse in childhood report prior periods when they did not remember the abuse. Herman and Schatzow (1987) reported "severe memory deficits" for abuse in 28% of their clinical sample of women in group therapy for incest survivors. Approximately two-thirds of their sample (64%) reported some degree of "amnesia." Briere and Conte (1993) found that 59% of 450 women and men in treatment for sexual abuse reported that, at some time before age 18, they had forgotten the sexual abuse they endured during childhood. Loftus et al. (1994b) reported that a sizable minority (31%) of their sample of sexually abused women in treatment for substance abuse had at least partial forgetting or incomplete memory of their abuse, and 19% reported prior periods of total lack of recall of the abuse. Gold et al. (1994) reported that 30% of patients in outpatient psychotherapy for treatment of the traumatic effects of childhood sexual abuse claimed to have previously completely blocked out any recollection of the abuse for a year or more. These studies and many others now appearing in the published literature indicate that a significant minority of victims of child sexual abuse in treatment report prior periods of forgetting.

Even in nonclinical samples of adults, a high rate of prior periods of forgetting childhood sexual abuse is reported. Among a national sample of psychologists, Feldman-Summers and Pope (1994) found that of the 79 participants who experienced childhood sexual abuse, 40% reported that they could not remember some or all of their abuse during an earlier period. D. M. Elliott ("Traumatic Events: Prevalence and Delayed Recall in the General Population," unpublished manuscript, Harbor-UCLA Medical Center, 1995) conducted a study of a national, stratified, random sample of 505 women and men. Of the sample, 23% reported a history of childhood sexual abuse, and, of these, 20% reported a time when they had no memory of this event, and an additional 22% reported a time when they had less memory of this event than they did at the time of the interview.

It has been suggested that rather than providing evidence of false negatives, the fact that many respondents from clinical samples report prior periods of forgetting may simply be attributable to false positives. The argument is that these respondents' "memories" of abuse may have been recovered under the influence of therapists who believe that amnesia for sexual abuse is common. However, no evidence is found in the studies of clinical samples that most of the memories were recovered by therapy. It is perhaps more feasible that if prior periods of forgetting or recently recovered memories of childhood sexual abuse are associated with higher rates of symptomatology (Elliott and Briere 1995), then we would expect those individuals who were sexually abused in childhood and who are currently in treatment for such symptomatology to have a higher rate of prior forgetting than those who are not in treatment. Studies that rely on community samples overcome problems associated with sampling bias and the possibility of an elevated rate of prior forgetting in clinical samples. Both community studies and clinical samples, however, used a retrospective methodology to gather information about forgetting of childhood sexual abuse and, as a result, are subject to the problem that such abuse is usually uncorroborated. In addition, studies must rely on retrospective accounts of prior forgetting, yet the validity of these accounts is unknown.

Finally, retrospective designs are unable to examine instances in which sexual abuse experienced in childhood continues to be forgotten. Obviously, researchers cannot survey adults and ask whether they were abused in childhood but have now forgotten. For this reason, two prospective-cohorts-design studies of child sexual abuse, in which abused and neglected children were followed up prospectively into adulthood, have received much attention.

Williams (1994) followed up women and men (Williams and Banyard 1996) who, in the early 1970s, were seen in a hospital emergency room for child sexual abuse and found that (17 years post abuse) 38% of the women (n = 129) and 55% of the men (n = 47) did not recall the abuse. Williams also reported that of the 80 women who recalled the documented abuse, 16% stated that there was a time in the past when they did not remember that it had happened to them. In a similar study, C. S. Widom ("Accuracy of adult reports of child abuse," unpublished manuscript, State University of New York at Albany, 1996) found that 32% of women (n = 70) and 58% of men (n = 19) with court-substantiated reports of child sexual victimization did not report such abuse on re-interview some 20 years later.

Neither study design called for directly confronting participants who appeared to have forgotten the abuse with the evidence of abuse documented in their records from the 1970s (a decision based on concern for protection of human subjects). It is, of course, possible that some of the interviewed men and women in these studies simply did not wish to talk about the abuse or were too embarrassed or ashamed to do so. Femina et al. (1990) reported that adolescents, when confronted with a failure to report a history of childhood physical abuse, indicated they were too ashamed or embarrassed to talk about it to the interviewer. Those investigators (Lindsay and Read 1994; Pope and Hudson 1995) who cite Femina et al. as evidence of deliberate nondisclosure fail to note that the Femina study was a follow-up of not only individuals who denied their abuse histories but also those who reported but minimized their abuse. The critical subsample in this study was also very small. In fact, only 8 of the 18 subjects who denied or minimized the documented abuse were recontacted for the clarification interview to determine whether they were deliberately denying the event or had actually forgotten it.

Williams (1994) contends that it is unlikely that embarrassment was the reason that so many women did not report the abuse in her study. Of the women who did not recall the child sexual abuse that brought them into the study (the "index" abuse), 68% told the interviewer about other sexual assaults (clearly involving different perpetrators and circumstances) that they experienced in childhood. Of the women who did recall the "index" abuse, the same proportion (68%) reported other incidents of child sexual abuse, indicating that those who did not recall the index abuse were no less likely to reveal details of other personal, upsetting, or potentially embarrassing experiences. The two prospective studies (C. S. Widom, "Accuracy of adult reports of child abuse," unpublished manuscript, State University of New York at Albany, 1996;

Williams 1994) have remarkably similar findings and are also consistent with the data from clinical samples. Although we cannot conclusively report what proportion of abuse victims forget, these studies suggest that a significant proportion of those with documented histories of sexual abuse in childhood, when reinterviewed as young adults, do not recall the abuse.

Mechanisms for forgetting child sexual abuse.   In earlier sections of this chapter, we reviewed some of the literature on memory and the mechanisms that may play a role in remembering or forgetting traumatic experiences. If many abuse survivors forget experiences of childhood sexual abuse or report periods of not remembering, what evidence do we have about the mechanisms for such forgetting? Various explanations are likely. Clinicians and researchers who have suggested that the findings from these studies provide evidence for certain theories about the actual mechanisms for the forgetting have been harshly criticized (Loftus and Ketcham 1994; Loftus et al. 1994a; Pope and Hudson 1995). These critics suggest that deliberate nondisclosure, allegations of amnesia for secondary gain (Pope and Hudson 1995), and normal forgetting (Loftus et al. 1994a) account for the "lack of recall" in these studies. They argue against any specific psychological mechanisms associated with abuse or other forms of traumatic stress. However, there is a growing body of scientific evidence on the psychological effects and memories of abuse (Briere and Conte 1993; Elliott and Briere 1995; Herman and Schatzow 1987) and clinical literature on survivors of child sexual abuse (see, for example, Briere 1992; Herman 1992; Terr 1988, 1990, 1991; van der Kolk and Fisler 1995) that provides support for trauma theory, which suggests that forgetting abuse reflects the use of psychological mechanisms such as cognitive avoidance, dissociation, and repression as coping strategies for the psychological distress associated with prior traumatic events.

In several studies, young age at the time of abuse has been associated with prior periods of forgetting (Briere and Conte 1993; Elliott, unpublished data, 1995; Herman and Schatzow 1987; Williams 1994). Although infantile amnesia and cognitive developmental processes could explain the forgetting by the youngest victims, several studies have documented such forgetting even among those who were older at the time of victimization (C. S. Widom, "Accuracy of Adult Reports of Child Abuse," unpublished manuscript, State University of New York at Albany, 1996; Williams 1994). Certainly, in some cases, the abuse may not be remembered because it was not very important, and a long time has passed. In cases of relatively less dramatic experiences, especially in people whose lives are full of other traumatic events, an episode or two of sexual touching by someone unimportant may simply be forgotten.

Clinical literature on adult survivors of child sexual abuse suggests that the aversiveness of the experience may lead some victims to engage in active strategies to avoid reminders of traumatic events and ultimately memories of the event. Over time, coping mechanisms may cause the experience to recede until it is accessible only with certain stimuli (Briere 1992). Both Briere and Conte (1993) and Herman and Schatzow (1987) found that, among their treatment-seeking respondents, having a prior period of no recall of the abuse was associated with *more violent episodes* of abuse and *younger age at the time of the abuse.* Herman and Schatzow suggested that massive repression was the main defensive resource available to their patients who were sexually and/or violently abused in early childhood. Briere and Conte suggested that the association they found between no recall and *trauma* (as measured by violence or injury) and the lack of association between no recall and *conflict* (as measured by guilt, shame, and enjoyment) fit better with the process of dissociation than with an active defensive process of repression. Similarly, Terr (1991) suggested that what she calls type II traumas (long-standing or repeated ordeals) may be more likely to result in denial and dissociation. Briere and Conte suggested that young age is associated with no recall for the abuse because younger children may be more likely to experience abuse as violent, thus motivating repression or dissociation, or may have fewer psychological defenses available to them other than forgetting. As evidence that the age–no recall association is not primarily attributable to cognitive developmental features of young children, Briere and Conte (1993) and Herman and Schatzow (1987) emphasized that many of their subjects who retrieved memories were very young at the time of abuse. Williams (1995) reported that those in her sample with recovered memories were on average 3 years younger at the time of abuse than those who reported continuous recollection of their abuse experiences.

In addition, memories of sexual abuse may be encoded, stored, and retrieved differently from other memories (van der Kolk and Fisler 1995), especially when the abuse occurs under circumstances of high arousal, terror, and extreme ambivalence; when escape is impossible; or when the meaning of the abuse, if confronted, could be devastating. The concepts of repression or dissociation as psychologically motivated defenses against knowing cannot be dismissed. Although the mechanisms that might explain such phenomena have not yet been confirmed in laboratory studies, this does not make them impossible.

In contrast to these findings, Williams (1994) reported that after controlling for age, no relationship was found between force used in the abuse and recall. On the other hand, the women in Williams's (1994) study who had been abused by someone with whom they had a closer relationship, a variable often associated with greater psychological distress, were more likely to have forgotten the abuse, even when abuse severity and age at time of abuse were controlled. Williams (1995) also

---

found that women in her sample who recalled the abuse but reported prior periods of forgetting were more likely than women who reported continuous memories of the abuse to have had weak or no support from their mothers. These findings are consistent with Freyd's (1994) notion of betrayal trauma.

Even though none of the studies discussed in this section delineates the specific mechanisms for the forgetting, the findings do suggest that in some individuals, the lack of recall of the abuse is based on more than just ordinary forgetting associated with the passage of time, their young age when abused, or a lack of salience of the event. Indeed, there is some reason to believe that the process of forgetting childhood sexual abuse may differ from that of forgetting other traumatic events of childhood. After all, most child sexual abuse occurs in secret. The sexual contact may be associated with shame and guilt, and the responses of others who learn about the abuse often do little to ensure comfort and unconflicted memories of the event, because their responses often convey shock, disbelief, and denial (Berliner and Conte 1990; Browne and Finkelhor 1986). However, one important study (Elliott, unpublished data, 1995) suggested that such forgetting or delayed recall is not limited to sexual abuse. Elliott found that the phenomenon occurs across a variety of traumas and is most likely with particularly traumatic events. Because any examination of memories of traumatic events can only rely on observed behavior, we may never have conclusive proof that a specific mechanism is responsible for the observable forgetting. Nevertheless, the variables found to be associated with forgetting in the studies to date are consistent with the hypothesis that complex psychological processes affect memories of childhood sexual abuse.

False Reports, Beliefs, or Memory—False Positives

Investigators have suggested that estimates of the prevalence of child sexual abuse in community surveys are inflated by false reports (Grossman and Pressley 1994; Lindsay and Read 1995; Loftus et al. 1994b), but no empirical evidence has been accumulated to describe how frequently such false positives actually occur, and no information is available that would allow reasonable estimates of the magnitude of the problem. Research on fictitious reports of abuse by children or their parents suggests a fabrication rate of 4%–8% (for review, see Everson and Boat 1989), and 2% of the women in Williams's (1994) study reported that they or others had fabricated the report of child sexual abuse. However, there is no evidence that fabrication occurs at even this rate when adults are asked behaviorally specific questions about whether they were sexually abused in childhood. No scientific evidence shows that adults commonly make purely fabricated allegations of abuse in childhood when surveyed using standard victimization screening techniques. This frequently raised issue will remain only theoretical until specific research is done to assess its frequency.

The body of research on false positives has focused on the issue of suggestibility and recovered memories of abuse (Kihlstrom 1993; Lindsay and Read 1994; Loftus 1993) and therapists' use of techniques designed to recover such memories. Several books and articles have made claims that a majority of therapists will, on occasion, hunt for repressed memories and will use suggestive techniques to do so (Ofshe and Watters 1993; Poole et al. 1995; Yapko 1994). Poole et al. (1995) surveyed American and British psychologists and concluded that 25% of therapists believe that recovering memories of abuse is an important part of therapy, believe they can identify patients with hidden memories during the initial session, and toward this end use two or more techniques (such as age regression or dream interpretation) to help patients recover memories of child sexual abuse (Poole et al. 1995). The critique of these practices (Lindsay and Read 1994) has grown out of and is supported by a tradition of laboratory research by cognitive psychologists on the fallibility of memory.

A profusion of research on suggestibility and memory shows that memory is reconstructive and imperfect (Loftus and Loftus 1980; Spence 1984), that memory can be influenced and distorted (Dodson and Johnson 1993), that confabulation can occur to fill in memory gaps, and that subjects can be persuaded to believe they heard, saw, or experienced events that they have not (Johnson et al. 1988, 1993; Lindsay 1994). Inaccurate memories can be strongly believed and convincingly described (Winograd and Neisser 1992). Much of the laboratory research on suggestibility of memory has involved paradigms in which individuals view an item or event (e.g., the presence of a barn in a photograph or the speed of a vehicle before an accident), are later given incorrect information about the event, and, finally, are asked about what they saw. Individuals who are given incorrect information are likely to incorporate that information into later reports of their memories of the event. This process is termed the *misinformation effect,* and it is argued that this effect also applies to memories of childhood sexual abuse. Some researchers assert that similar processes may lead to a patient's false belief that he or she was sexually abused if such a history is suggested by a therapist (see Lindsay and Read 1994).

Criticisms of the application of laboratory research to investigations of memory of childhood sexual abuse have focused on the ecological validity of the studies—that is, its applicability to the real-world experience of child molestation and its aftermath (Berliner and Williams 1994). Just because an experimenter can make a person think that she or he saw a barn in a bucolic country scene when there was no barn, it does not necessarily mean that someone can be made to falsely believe that she or he was sexually abused when, in fact, the abuse did not occur. Changing or adding a feature to an event, as is the procedure in much of the laboratory research, is not the same as making someone believe that an entirely new event occurred (Olio 1994; Pezdek 1995). In addition, implanting memories for traumatic events and for self-referent events may be a very different matter. Self-involved memories may be less susceptible to the misinformation effect. Of course, research ethics preclude any experiment that would attempt to implant memories of something as serious as sexual abuse.

Recently, several studies have attempted to directly assess the implantation of memories for events that would be traumatic had they occurred, to examine types of events that are more likely to be implanted, and to investigate the factors associated with successful implantation of memories for events that did not occur. Several paradigms have been used, but all have in common an attempt to make younger family members of the researchers' collaborators "remember" events that did not occur. A "lost in a shopping mall" study (Loftus and Pickrell 1995) found that 25% of the adults ($n = 24$) could lead a child or other relative to believe that he or she had been lost in a shopping mall when he or she was 5 years old. Five of the six participants in this study who "remembered" the false event also generated additional details about the incident.

Hyman et al. (1995) attempted to address criticisms that the shopping mall study tests for a "memory" of a universally feared, high-base-rate childhood event (separation from a parent) by asking college students about their memories of false events that were more unusual, such as attending a wedding and knocking over a punch bowl or having to evacuate a grocery store when a sprinkler system was accidentally activated. None of the 51 subjects had false recalls during the first interview, but 25% (13) claimed to recall these events by the third interview (more information and increasing demands for recall were provided with each reinterview). In another study, Pezdek (1995) tested the hypothesis that it would be easier to implant memories for events for which one has a generic script. She used two false events that differed in the availability of scripts: 1) the familiar event—getting lost and 2) the unfamiliar event—receiving an enema. Pezdek found that 3 of the 20 participants remembered the familiar event, whereas none of the 20 participants remembered the unfamiliar event. Pezdek concluded that events will be suggestively implanted to the extent that the suggested event is familiar.

This research suggests that individuals can be made to believe that they had experiences that did not actually occur, but they are more resistant to the implantation of memories for events that are less familiar. I. E. Hyman and F. G. Billings ("Individual Differences and the Creation of False Childhood Memories," unpublished manuscript, Western Washington University, 1995) found that those who created false memories scored higher on measures of dissociation and creative imagination, suggesting that one's ability to engage in reality monitoring is related to acceptance of false events. Hyman and Pentland (1996) reported that individuals who were asked to form a mental image of an event and to describe it to an interviewer were more likely to create a false event. Interestingly, they were also more likely to recover memories of a previously unavailable true event.

It must be kept in mind that all of these studies involved fairly small samples and that most participants resisted implanted memory. It is unclear whether an actual memory is in fact recalled or whether it was created in response to the demand characteristics of the experiment (e.g., active confirmation of the truth of the experience by an older family member who claimed to have been present).

How generalizable these findings are to issues of false positives in cases of child sexual abuse is unclear. The demand characteristics of these experiments in which an older, more powerful adult directly asserts that the event took place, claims to have been present, and asks the individual to try hard to remember do not describe the demand characteristics of most therapy. If, however, such pressures were placed on a patient to remember childhood sexual abuse, subsequent recollections, although not necessarily untrue (Hyman and Pentland 1996), would be suspect. These findings have important implications for clinical practice, which are discussed below.

Remembering Childhood Sexual Abuse—True Positives

Taking the position that some women are amnesic for sexual abuse that happened in childhood does not mean that all or even most victims forget. Most individuals who were molested after the offset of infantile amnesia probably have continuous memories of the abuse (Terr 1988; Williams 1994). This does not mean that individuals remember every detail of the abuse experience nor that they remember it every waking hour, but they recall that it happened. Indeed, for some, the memories are all too vivid.

Williams (1994) found that 62% of the women and 45% of the men in her sample (Williams and Banyard 1996) recalled abuse that had been documented in their hospital records in childhood. Of the women who recalled the abuse, 84% reported that memories of the abuse had been continuous (Williams 1995). Williams was able to compare the accounts of adult women with the details of the abuse recorded in the 1970s and, therefore, was also able to examine an important subset of those who remembered their abuse—those who currently remembered their abuse but who had some prior period of forgetting. The experiences of these women can help us understand the variability of memory even among the true positive group and how complicated it is to distinguish between false positives and true positives.

Williams (1995) found that women with recovered memories were younger at the time of abuse than those who had continuous memories of the experience. Although the number of women in this sample with recovered memories of abuse was small ($n = 12$) and the findings must be treated as preliminary, this study suggests that women who report prior forgetting are able to recall the abuse. Although the women's reports of some details changed, their accounts of the abuse were surprisingly clear and true to the basic elements of the original incident. Interestingly, despite few gross inaccuracies, the women with recovered memories were often very unsure about their memories and made statements such as, "What I remember is mostly from a dream" or "I'm really not too sure about this." The woman's level of uncertainty about recovered memories was not associated with more inaccuracies in her account. In fact, the accounts of the women who reported their memories to be vague were no more inaccurate than those who reported their memories to be clear. This suggests that individuals who are recalling true events may be relatively unsure about these memories. Lack of clarity about abuse experiences, particularly those that occurred at a young age, should not be seen as evidence that the events did not occur. Of course, these findings cannot be used to assert the validity of *all* recovered memories of child abuse, but they do suggest that recovered memories of childhood sexual abuse reported by adults can be quite accurate.

Memory and Symptomatology

The previous sections provide some support for the notion that childhood sexual abuse can be forgotten, although the mechanisms that cause such memory lapses are much less clear. An important next question pertains to the mental health consequences of such forgetting. Theories that address this issue are closely linked to discussions of mechanisms that underlie the forgetting. For example, if we believe that survivors, such as those in Williams's study (1994) who did not report having been abused, either choose not to report their history or had forgotten the incident as a result of normal forgetting processes, then we might speculate that their mental health outcomes would not be significantly different from those of survivors who report continuous recall of their abuse. On the other hand, if we theorize that the forgetting is related to an avoidance coping style that may in some instances be adaptive (Tromp et al. 1995), then perhaps survivors with no reported memory for the abuse will actually have a better mental health outcome. Finally, if we follow theories that suggest that forgetting of trauma is a result of repression, dissociation, or physiological alterations in neurochemistry caused by extreme stress, then we would predict that individuals with memory problems would report higher levels of psychological symptomatology (Briere and Conte 1993; Herman 1992; Spiegel 1986; van der Kolk and Fisler 1995). Preliminary results from several studies raise more questions than they answer and suggest that some combination of these anticipated results may be expected.

Williams and Banyard (1995) have presented some preliminary exploratory analyses of the effects of remembering on mental health symptoms. Participants in the prospective study were divided into two groups: those who had continuous recall of their sexual abuse and those who either did not currently remember or reported some period in the past when they did not remember. The groups were further divided based on their age at the time of the index abuse. The investigators hypothesized few differences would be found between subjects with and without memory problems who were young (9 years or younger) at the time of the abuse. A variety of mechanisms for forgetting might have been operating in this group, including the effects of childhood amnesia and other developmental interferences, making clear patterns of effects difficult to discern. On the other hand, the investigators hypothesized that those who were ages 10, 11, or 12 at the time of the abuse but did not remember it or had some prior period of forgetting would have more mental health symptoms if a mechanism such as repression or dissociation was at work. The study produced limited conclusions. Small sample sizes contributed to a lack of overall significance in the analyses. However, a descriptive examination of the magnitude of differences among the various groups showed a trend in the expected direction, with those participants who were older at the time of the abuse and had memory problems also reporting higher levels of sexual abuse trauma symptoms such as fear of men or sexual problems.

Studies by Briere and Conte (1993) and Elliott and Briere (1995) also address this issue. Briere and Conte studied a sample of 450 adults who had been sexually abused as children and were in treatment at the time of the study. They found that those individuals who did not have continuous recall of their abuse, but had some prior period of forgetting, also had higher scores on the General Symptom Index of the Symptom Checklist—90 (SCL-90). Elliott and Briere expanded this work and examined differences among sexual abuse survivors who had continuous recall of their abuse, those who had some prior period of forgetting but recovered the memory of their abuse very recently (less than 2 years before the interview), and those who had recovered memories more than 2 years before the research interview. Their results indicated that those individuals with more recent recall of their abuse reported the highest levels of symptomatology such as posttraumatic intrusion, avoidance, dissociation, and the highest scores on measures of posttraumatic stress. They discussed these findings as evidence that the process of recovering memories may produce a resurgence in posttraumatic symptoms, and individuals experiencing this phenomenon may require additional clinical support. They also highlighted the fact that such symptoms seem to abate over time, as evidenced by the lower rates of distress reported by the remote recall group. Elliott and Briere suggested that the increased symptoms associated with recall may be distressing, but they may also help to facilitate the healing process. This theory may support work by Pennebaker (1982, 1990), who discussed the curative effects of disclosing and discussing traumatic events rather than inhibiting their discussion or ruminating about them in silence. Such events can be discussed only if they are remembered.

This area of study requires much future research. Some data will come from studies that clarify the mechanisms that may produce amnesia for child sexual abuse in some individuals, whereas others have frequent intrusive flashbacks. Indeed, perhaps as we discover the variety of mechanisms that may lead to forgetting, we will have a better understanding of the full range of outcomes associated with this response. We may never be able to conclude that forgetting is either adaptive or problematic and may find that it can be either or both for any particular individual; also, it may vary in effect at different stages of the life course. Although Pennebaker (1982) emphasized the benefits of discussing traumatic experiences, he also cited evidence that in some cases, putting the experience behind one and finding the ability to not dwell on it may be very adaptive. We need to learn much more about the conditions under which forgetting sexual abuse may be adaptive and the conditions under which it may create difficulties.

Research Implications

Laboratory research indicates many reasons to be concerned about the accuracy of memories of childhood sexual abuse. These include the fallibility of memory and the passage of time. However, the concepts of source misattributions and misinformation effect could also be applied to studies designed to understand the false negatives and to explain the memory processes that could be involved in total amnesia for abuse or in false beliefs or false memories about an event (such as when a young woman misremembers actual sexual abuse only as an injury to her genitals caused by a fall from a bicycle or when a young man recalls his actual abuse as a consensual experience with an older woman). Problems of source monitoring, an influential interviewer, an interviewer seeking to confirm preconceived ideas, and repeated or persistent suggestion could result in false positives *or* false negatives.

Research studies designed to examine how the dynamics of sexual abuse, particularly abuse by a close, powerful family member, may contribute to the creation of false beliefs of nonabuse would be useful. Future research could examine what happens when subjects are encouraged or pressured to forget and the extent to which false memories of true events are influenced by fears and posttraumatic stress disorder; by feelings of guilt, shame, or betrayal; or by reframing an event to a more socially and personally acceptable scenario. Just as the social context can distort memory in the direction of falsely believing one was abused, it seems reasonable that it can distort memory in the direction of dissociation and forgetting.

Our review of the research suggests other interesting questions for future research: What accounts for forgetting some parts versus all of the abuse? What accounts for short periods versus long periods of forgetting? What accounts for complete lack of recall and never remembering the abuse? What is the association between such patterns of recall and social and psychological functioning in adulthood? These and other questions about the phenomenology and mechanism of forgetting about childhood sexual abuse and other childhood trauma require further study. Longitudinal research is needed to examine what happens to memory in childhood and throughout the life span.

The field of child abuse and neglect, in general, and child sexual abuse, in particular, would also benefit from well-designed treatment outcome studies (Finkelhor and Berliner 1995), including studies of the use and effect of techniques of memory recovery. Clinical research should also focus on not only the impact of memory on symptomatology but also the impact of false memories or beliefs of abuse on the individual and the family.

Treatment Implications

Although an assessment of the treatment issues in the area of memory for childhood sexual abuse is beyond the scope of this chapter, a number of important treatment implications emerge from this research review (for discussion of some treatment issues, see Bowman and Mertz 1996; Enns et al. 1995). Researchers who study the fallibility of memory and those advocates who are concerned with the problems of false positives have raised important questions for professionals who work with trauma survivors. Others have raised serious questions about the use of active memory recovery strategies that may lead to the development of false memories or false beliefs that one was abused when, in fact, no such abuse occurred. Surveys of clinical practitioners indicate that some clinicians need more information about normal memory processes and could benefit from specific guidance about potential problems of suggestibility and memories of childhood sexual abuse.

Although it is not easy to implant memories for events about which an individual is unfamiliar and it is not clear how generalizable the research is to memories of childhood sexual abuse, laboratory research indicates that false beliefs about childhood experiences can be generated by pressing for a memory, especially when the individual has a ready script available for that experience (Pezdek 1995) or when the individual is asked to form a mental image of an event and to describe it to an interviewer.

One interesting implication of Pezdek's findings is that those who were truly abused may also be more susceptible to false beliefs about abuse because these individuals have a ready script for child sexual abuse available. On the other hand, evidence from Hyman and Pentland (1996) indicates that techniques such as guided imagery may assist with recall of memories of previously forgotten true events. These paradoxical findings from laboratory research suggest that clinicians must proceed with caution in working with patients' memories of abuse and in drawing conclusions about abuse histories. However, the standards of proof or necessity for corroboration of any memory of a childhood event will vary for individual, therapeutic, and criminal justice or other legal system decision making (Bowman and Mertz 1996).

These cautions must be balanced by the research on the problem of false negatives, which has implied that it would be unwise and possibly harmful for therapists or others to dismiss patients' recollections of abuse simply because the memories are vague. Findings from Williams's (1995) study support the idea that when previously forgotten sexual abuse experiences are subsequently recalled, they contain many of the characteristics of remembering noted in clinical settings. The women's memories came not from therapy, but through environmentally triggered cues (see also Elliott, unpublished data, 1995). The women reported a gradual process of remembering, often initially characterized by vague and fragmentary images. Many said that these images were contained in dreams. Although the women who recovered memories were often not very confident about their memories, when their accounts of the abuse were compared with earlier documentation of abuse, they were accurate—as reliable as those of the women who had always remembered their abuse. Research on the experiences of those in the true positive group has verified that child sexual abuse has a wide range of negative consequences. Clinicians cannot afford to collude with families and society in silencing survivors' recollections of their abuse. Because knowledge of the effect of child sexual abuse on memory remains very limited, we must conduct more research to better understand this phenomenon and combine such research with an ongoing discussion of its implications for practitioners.

References

Andrews B, Morton J, Bekerian DA, et al: The recovery of memories in clinical practice: experiences and beliefs of British Psychological Society practitioners. The Psychologist, May 1995, pp 209–214

Beckett K: Culture and the politics of signification: the case of child sexual abuse. Social Problems 43(1):57–76, 1996

Beitchman JH, Zucker KJ, DaCosta GA, et al: A review of the long-term effects of child sexual abuse. Child Abuse Negl 16:101–118, 1992

Belli RF, Loftus EF: Recovered memories of childhood abuse: a source monitoring perspective, in Dissociation: Theory, Clinical, and Research Perspectives. Edited by Lynn SJ, Rhue JW. New York, Guilford, 1994, pp 415–433

Berliner L, Conte JR: The process of victimization: the victim's perspective. Child Abuse Negl 14:29–40, 1990

Berliner L, Loftus E: Sexual abuse accusations: desperately seeking reconciliation. Journal of Interpersonal Violence 7:570–578, 1992

Berliner L, Williams LM: Memories of child sexual abuse: response to Lindsay and Read. Journal of Applied Cognitive Psychology 8:379–387, 1994

Bowman CG, Mertz E: A dangerous direction: legal intervention in sexual abuse survivor therapy. Harvard Law Review 109:549–639, 1996

Bremner JD, Krystal JH, Southwick SM, et al: Functional neuroanatomical correlates of the effects of stress on memory. J Trauma Stress 8:527–554, 1995

Brewin CR, Andrews B, Gotlib IH: Psychopathology and early experience: a reappraisal of retrospective reports. Psychol Bull 113:82–98, 1993

Briere J: Child Abuse Trauma: Theory and Treatment of the Lasting Effects. Newbury Park, CA, Sage, 1992

Briere J, Conte J: Self-reported amnesia for abuse in adults molested as children. J Trauma Stress 6:21–31, 1993

Briere J, Zaidi LY: Sexual abuse histories and sequelae in female psychiatric emergency room patients. Am J Psychiatry 146:1602–1606, 1989

Brown R, Kulik J: Flashbulb memories. Cognition 5:73–99, 1977

Browne A, Finkelhor D: The impact of child sexual abuse: a review of the research. Psychol Bull 99:66–77, 1986

Burke A, Heuer F, Reisberg D: Remembering emotional events. Memory and Cognition 20:277–290, 1992

Cahill L, Brins B, Weber M, et al: β-Adrenergic activation and memory for emotional events. Nature 371:702–704, 1994

Carlson EB (ed): Trauma Research Methodology. Lutherville, MD, Sidran Press, 1996

Ceci SJ, Caves RD, Howe MJA: Children's long-term memory for information that is incongruous with their prior knowledge. Br J Psychol 72:443–450, 1981

Conte J, Wolfe S, Smith T: What sexual offenders tell us about prevention strategies. Child Abuse Negl 13:293–301, 1989

Courtois CA: The memory retrieval process in incest survivor therapy. Journal of Child Sexual Abuse 1:15–31, 1992

Dodson CS, Johnson MK: Rate of false source attributions depends on how questions are asked. Am J Psychol 106:451–557, 1993

Elliott DM, Briere J: Posttraumatic stress associated with delayed recall of sexual abuse: a general population study. J Trauma Stress 8:629–648, 1995

Enns CZ, McNeilly CL, Corkery JM, et al: The debate about delayed memories of child sexual abuse: a feminist perspective. The Counseling Psychologist 23:181–279, 1995

Everson M, Boat B: False allegations of sexual abuse by children and adolescents. J Am Acad Child Adolesc Psychiatry 28:230–235, 1989

Feldman-Summers S, Pope KS: The experience of "forgetting" childhood abuse: a national survey of psychologists. J Consult Clin Psychol 62:636–639, 1994

Femina DD, Yeager CA, Lewis DO: Child abuse: adolescent records vs. adult recall. Child Abuse Negl 14:227–231, 1990

Finkelhor D: Sexually Victimized Children. New York, Free Press, 1979

Finkelhor D, Berliner L: Research on the treatment of sexually abused children. J Am Acad Child Adolesc Psychiatry 34:1408–1423, 1995

Fivush R, Hammond NR: Autobiographical memory across the preschool years: toward reconceptualizing childhood amnesia, in Knowing and Remembering in Young Children. Edited by Fivush R, Hudson JA. New York, Cambridge University Press, 1990, pp 223–248

Fivush R, Reese E: The social construction of autobiographical memory, in Theoretical Perspectives on Autobiographical Memory. Edited by Conway MA, Rubin DC, Spinnler H, et al. Boston, MA, Kluwer Academic Press, 1992, pp 115–132

Fivush R, Schwartzmueller A: Say it once again: effects of repeated questions on children's event recall. J Trauma Stress 8:555–580, 1995

Freud S: The Standard Edition of the Complete Psychological Works of Sigmund Freud, Vol 7. Translated and edited by Strachey J. London, Hogarth Press, 1953

Freyd JJ: Betrayal trauma: traumatic amnesia as an adaptive response to childhood abuse. Ethics and Behavior 4:307–329, 1994

Gold SN, Hughes D, Hohnecker L: Degrees of repression of sexual abuse memories. Am Psychol 49:441–442, 1994

Goodman GS, Quas JA, Batterman-Faunce JM, et al: Predictors of accurate and inaccurate memories of traumatic events experienced in childhood. Consciousness and Cognition 3:269–294, 1994

Grossman LR, Pressley M: Introduction. Applied Cognitive Psychology 8:277–280, 1994

Hartman CR, Burgess AW: Information processing of trauma. Child Abuse Negl 17:47–58, 1993

Henry B, Moffitt TE, Caspi A, et al: On the "remembrance of things past": a longitudinal evaluation of the retrospective method. Psychological Assessment 6:92–101, 1994

Herman JL: Trauma and Recovery. New York, Basic Books, 1992

Herman JL, Schatzow E: Recovery and verification of memories of childhood sexual trauma. Psychoanalytic Psychology 4:1–14, 1987

Howe ML, Courage ML: On resolving the enigma of infantile amnesia. Psychol Bull 113:305–326, 1993

Howe ML, Courage ML, Peterson C: How can I remember when "I" wasn't there: long-term retention of traumatic experiences and emergence of the cognitive self. Consciousness and Cognition 3:327–355, 1994

Hyman IE, Pentland J: The role of mental imagery in the creation of false childhood memories. Journal of Memory and Language 35:101–117, 1996

Hyman IE, Husband TH, Billings FJ: False memories of childhood experiences. Applied Cognitive Psychology 9:181–197, 1995

Johnson MK, Foley MA, Suengas AG, et al: Phenomenal characteristics of memories for perceived and imagined autobiographical events. J Exp Psychol Gen 4:371–376, 1988

Johnson MK, Hashtroude S, Lindsay DS: Source monitoring. Psychol Bull 114:3–28, 1993

Kihlstrom JF: The recovery of memory in the laboratory and clinic. Paper presented at the joint convention of Rocky Mountain Psychological Association and Western Psychological Association, Phoenix, AZ, April 1993

Koss MP, Tromp S, Tharan M: Traumatic memories: empirical foundations, forensic and clinical implications. Clinical Psychology Scientific Practice 2(2):111–132, 1995

Kramer TH, Buckhout R, Fox P, et al: Effects of stress on recall. Applied Cognitive Psychology 5:483–488, 1991

Leippe M, Manion A, Romanczyk A: Eyewitness memory for a touching experience: accuracy differences between child and adult witnesses. Journal of Applied Cognitive Psychology 76:367–379, 1991

Lindsay DS: Memory source monitoring and eyewitness testimony, in Adult Eyewitness Testimony: Current Trends and Developments. Edited by Lindsay DC. New York, Cambridge University Press, 1994, pp 27–55

Lindsay DS, Read JD: Psychotherapy and memories of childhood sexual abuse: a cognitive perspective. Applied Cognitive Psychology 8:281–338, 1994

Lindsay DS, Read JD: "Memory work" and recovered memories of childhood sexual abuse: scientific evidence and public, professional, and personal issues. Psychology, Public Policy, and Law 1:846–908, 1995

Loftus EF: The reality of repressed memories. Am Psychol 48:518–537, 1993

Loftus EF: Remembering dangerously. Skeptical Inquirer. March/April, 1995, pp 20–29

Loftus EF, Burns TE: Mental shock can produce retrograde amnesia. Memory and Cognition 10:318–323, 1982

Loftus EF, Christianson S: Malleability of memory for emotional events, in Aversion, Avoidance, and Anxiety. Edited by Archer T, Nilsson L. Hillsdale, NJ, Lawrence Erlbaum, 1989, pp 311–322

Loftus EF, Davies GM: Distortions in the memory of children. Journal of Social Issues 40:51–67, 1984

Loftus EF, Ketcham K: The Myth of Repressed Memories. New York, St Martin's Press, 1994

Loftus EF, Loftus GR: On the permanence of stored information in the human brain. Am Psychol 35:409–420, 1980

Loftus EF, Pickrell JE: The formation of false memories. Psychiatric Annals 25:720–725, 1995

Loftus EF, Smith KD, Klinger MR, et al: Memory and mismemory for health events, in Questions About Questions: Inquiries Into the Cognitive Bases of Surveys. Edited by Tanur JM. New York, Russell Sage Foundation, 1992, pp 102–137

Loftus EF, Garry M, Feldman J: Forgetting sexual trauma: what does it mean when 38% forget? J Consult Clin Psychol 62:1177–1181, 1994a

Loftus EF, Polonsky S, Fullilove MT: Memories of childhood sexual abuse: remembering and repressing. Psychology of Women Quarterly 18:67–84, 1994b

McHugh PR: Reconciliation: scientific, clinical and legal issues of false memory syndrome. Conference Opening Remarks, Memory and Reality. Baltimore, MD, December 1994

Nadel L, Zola-Morgan S: Infantile amnesia: a neurological perspective, in Infant Memory: Its Relation to Normal and Pathological Memory in Humans and Other Animals. Edited by Moscovitch M. New York, Plenum, 1984, pp 145–172

Neimark J: The diva of disclosure: memory researcher Elizabeth Loftus. Psychology Today 29(1):48, 1996

Nelson K: The ontogeny of memory for real events, in Remembering Reconsidered: Ecological and Traditional Approaches to the Study of Memory. Edited by Neisser U, Winograd E. New York, Cambridge University Press, 1988, pp 244–276

Nelson K, Ross G: The generalities and specifics of long-term memory in infants and young children, in New Directions for Child Development: Children's Memory. Edited by Perlmutter M. San Francisco, CA, Jossey-Bass, 1980, pp 87–101

Ofshe RJ, Watters E: Making monsters. Society 3(3):4–16, 1993

Olio KA: Truth in memory. Am Psychol 49:442–443, 1994

Pennebaker JW: The Psychology of Physical Symptoms. New York, Springer Verlag, 1982

Pennebaker JW: Opening Up, the Healing Power of Confiding in Others. New York, William Morrow, 1990

Pezdek K: What types of false childhood memories are not likely to be suggestively planted? Paper presented at the meeting of the Psychonomic Society, Los Angeles, CA, November 1995

Pillemer DB, White SH: Childhood events recalled by children and adults. Adv Child Dev Behav 21:297–340, 1989

Poole DA, Lindsay DS, Memon A, et al: Psychotherapy and the recovery of memories of childhood sexual abuse: doctoral-level therapists' beliefs, practices, and experiences. J Consult Clin Psychol 63:426–437, 1995

Pope HG, Hudson JI: Can individuals "repress" memories of childhood sexual abuse? An examination of the evidence. Psychiatric Annals 25:715–719, 1995

Rogers ML: Factors influencing recall of childhood sexual abuse. J Trauma Stress 8:691–716, 1995

Rubin D, Kozin M: Vivid memories. Cognition 16:81–95, 1984

Russell DEH: The Secret Trauma: Incest in the Lives of Girls and Women. New York, Basic Books, 1986

Saywitz KJ, Goodman GS, Nicholas E, et al: Children's memories of a physical examination involving genital touch: implications for reports of child sexual abuse. J Consult Clin Psychol 59:682–691, 1991

Schacter DL, Kagan J, Leichtman MD: True and false memories in children and adults: a cognitive neuroscience perspective. Psychology, Public Policy, and Law 1:411–428, 1995

Siegel DJ: Memory, trauma, and psychotherapy. Journal of Psychotherapy Practice and Research 4:93–122, 1995

Spence DP: Narrative Truth and Historical Truth. New York, WW Norton, 1984

Spiegel D: Dissociating damage. Am J Clin Hypn 29:123–131, 1986

Spiegel D: Functional disorders with memory aspects: impact of acute vs. chronic and recurrent trauma on memory. Conference on Memories of Trauma, Clark University, Worcester, MA, December 1993

Squire LR: On the course of forgetting in very long-term memory. J Exp Psychol 15:241–245, 1989

Terr L: What happens to early memories of trauma? A study of twenty children under age five at the time of documented traumatic events. J Am Acad Child Adolesc Psychiatry 27:96–104, 1988

Terr LC: Too Scared to Cry. New York, Harper & Row, 1990

Terr LC: Childhood traumas: an outline and overview. Am J Psychiatry 148:10–20, 1991

Tromp S, Koss MP, Figueredo AJ, et al: Are rape memories different? A comparison of rape, other unpleasant, and pleasant memories among employed women. J Trauma Stress 8:607–628, 1995

Usher JA, Neisser U: Childhood amnesia and the beginnings of memory for four early life events. J Exp Psychol Gen 122:155–165, 1993

van der Kolk BA: Biological considerations about emotions, trauma, memory, and the brain, in Human Feelings: Explorations Affect Development and Meaning. Edited by Brown A, Khantzian M. (in press)

van der Kolk BA, Fisler R: Dissociation and the fragmentary nature of traumatic memories: overview and exploratory study. J Trauma Stress 8:505–526, 1995

van der Kolk BA, van der Hart O: The intrusive past: the flexibility of memory and the engraving of trauma. American Image 48:425–454, 1991

Wakefield H, Underwager R: Recovered memories of alleged sexual abuse: lawsuits against parents. Behavioral Sciences and the Law 10:483–507, 1991

Williams LM: Recall of childhood trauma: a prospective study of women's memories of child sexual abuse. J Consult Clin Psychol 62:1167–1176, 1994

Williams LM: Recovered memories of abuse in women with documented child sexual victimization histories. J Trauma Stress 8:649–673, 1995

Williams LM, Banyard VL: Consequences of remembering for adult adjustment in female survivors of sexual abuse: a prospective study. Paper presented at the 4th International Family Violence Research Conference, Durham, NH, July 1995

Williams LM, Banyard VL: Childhood trauma: men's memories of child sexual abuse. Paper presented at the NATO Advanced Scientific Institute on Trauma and Memory, Port de Bourgenay, France, June 1996

Williams LM, Finkelhor D: Paternal caregiving and incest: a test of a biosocial model. Am J Orthopsychiatry 65:101–113, 1995

Winograd E, Neisser U: Affect and Accuracy in Recall: Studies of "Flashbulb" Memories. New York, Cambridge University Press, 1992

Yapko M: Suggestions of Abuse: True and False Memories of Childhood Sexual Trauma. New York, Simon & Schuster, 1994

Chapter 10

Repressed Memories in Patients With Dissociative Disorder: Literature Review, Controlled Study, and Treatment Recommendations

Philip M. Coons, M.D., Elizabeth S. Bowman, M.D., and Victor Milstein, Ph.D.

> Whereas some doctors never trouble their heads about traumatic memories and do not even know that these exist, and whereas others fancy them everywhere, there is a place for persons who take a middle course and who believe they are able to detect the existence of traumatic memories in specific cases. The doctors comprising the last group need diagnostic rules.
>
> *Janet (1925), quoted in Powell and Boer (1995, p. 1296)*

Currently, a heated controversy is raging among mental health professionals over whether memories of traumatic events can be forgotten and, if so, whether the process of forgetting should be called "repression," as has been the tradition since the time of Freud. Mental health professionals have become polarized into two groups. At one extreme are experimental psychologists (Ceci and Bruck 1993; Kihlstrom 1995; Lindsay and Read 1994; Loftus 1993; Spanos et al. 1994; Usher and Neisser 1993; Wakefield and Underwager 1992, 1994; Yapko 1994) and a few academic psychiatrists (Frankel 1994; McHugh and Butterfield 1993; Orne et al. 1988; Pope and Hudson 1995), who stress pseudomemory formation through the use of suggestive interview techniques, social pressure from self-help groups or overzealous therapists, hypnosis, dream analysis, and guided imagery. Experimental research in this area, unfortunately, has largely ignored the traumatized clinical population, and conclusions have been unfairly extrapolated from a largely nonclinical population of children and college students.

It is clear from this research, however, that memory is a reconstructive process (Spence 1995) and that many factors impinge on its accuracy. In a review of the literature on flashbacks, Frankel (1994) found that posttraumatic flashbacks may be considerably distorted compared with the actual traumatic event. Ceci and Bruck's review (1993) of the child literature indicates that the memory of children, especially young children, may be modified through suggestion, however subtle. Research on hypnotic recall indicates that memories may be created or distorted by the use of suggestive interview techniques and that individuals who have such "memories" may be extremely confident about their accuracy even after being told the truth (Orne et al. 1988).

At the other extreme are practicing mental health clinicians with years of clinical experience in treating victims of trauma. Until recently, many have been largely ignorant of the nature of memory and how the process of suggestion can distort memory retrieval. It is also unfortunate that until recently, neither group has paid sufficient attention to the other's scientific literature.

A large factor in creating the dispute over memories of abuse was the revision of many state laws to lengthen the statute of limitations for the recovery of damages due to childhood abuse. Many states now allow civil suits to be filed for damages when memories of childhood abuse finally surface, even if the victim is in her or his third, fourth, or fifth decade of life. This legal process has torn asunder many families and has been instrumental in the formation of the False Memory Syndrome Foundation, an organization composed of mostly parents who dispute their children's allegations of prior childhood abuse. This organization, which has many luminaries in the field of experimental memory research on its board of directors, has been behind an effort in several state legislatures to strictly limit how patients who allege memories of childhood abuse may be treated (Cronin 1995; Golston 1995).

The importance of this dispute cannot be underestimated. It essentially reiterates the same controversy that plagued Sigmund Freud and his colleagues and eventually led Freud to reverse his seduction hypothesis in favor of fantasy being responsible for the production of reports of sexual abuse in some of his patients (Powell and Boer 1995). This dispute has led seven journals to devote entire issues to the controversy (*Applied Cognitive Psychology* 1994; *Consciousness and Cognition* 1994, 1995; *Counseling Psychologist* 1995; *International Journal of Clinical and Experimental Hypnosis* 1994, 1995; *Journal of Psychohistory* 1995; *Journal of Traumatic Stress* 1995; *Psychiatric Annals* 1995) and several major organizations and prominent individuals to issue statements (American Medical Association, Council on Scientific Affairs 1994; American Psychiatric Association, Board of Trustees 1994; American Society of Clinical Hypnosis 1995; British Psychological Society 1995) and treatment guidelines (Allen 1995; Bloom 1994; Fowler 1994; Gutheil 1993;

Hammond 1995; Lynn and Nash 1994; van der Hart and Nijenhuis 1995; Watkins 1993; Yapko 1994) on the issue of memory and repression. Members of the American Psychological Association have become so mired in the dispute that their official statement is not expected until 1996. Conclusions of these major mental health organizations have been tempered by the relative lack of research in this important area. Most statements concur that memories of traumatic events can be forgotten but that pseudomemory formation is also possible. At present, the only way to determine whether a specific traumatic memory is genuine is with outside corroboration.

Review of Studies of Posttraumatic Memories

Studies Involving Predominantly Nonsexual Trauma

It is clear, even from the older literature, that memories of trauma can be forgotten and later retrieved. During World War II, several studies of amnesia for combat-related trauma were done (Table 10–1). Sargant and Slater (1941) found that 14% of 1,000 soldiers hospitalized for neuroses had amnesia. Torrie (1944) found a 9% incidence of amnesia and fugue in 1,000 cases of anxiety neuroses and hysteria among troops in North Africa. Henderson and Moore (1944) found a 5% incidence of amnesia among 200 neuropsychiatric patients in the South Pacific. Fisher (1944) observed and treated 20 sailors with fugue states. Although these studies had problems (i.e., neuropsychological causes for the amnesias were not ruled out in a consistent manner), it is remark-

Table 10–1. Studies of amnesia associated with combat during World War II

Study	Nature of population	Number in series	Percentage with amnesia	Confirmation of trauma
Sargant and Slater 1941	Soldiers hospitalized with neuroses	1,000	14	No
Torrie 1944	Soldiers with anxiety/hysteria	1,000	9	No
Henderson and Moore 1944	Soldiers with neuropsychiatric illness	200	5	No
Fisher 1944	Sailors with fugue	20	100	No

able that many amnesias cleared dramatically with the use of hypnosis, a result one would not expect if the cause were organic. Other major case reports of amnesia for trauma stem from other wars, including World War I (Thom and Fenton 1920), the Korean War (Archibald and Tuddenham 1956), the Vietnam War (Hendin et al. 1984; Sonneberg et al. 1985), and the Middle Eastern war between Israel and Egypt (Kalman 1977).

Both Jaffe (1968) and Niederland (1968) reported cases of amnesia among survivors of concentration camps, and Modai (1994) reported a case of amnesia in a Holocaust survivor who was not interned in a concentration camp. More recently, Kinzie (1993) reported amnesia in Southeast Asian war refugees.

Goldfield et al. (1988) reported on amnesia as a sequelae of torture. The experience of dissociative symptoms such as depersonalization, derealization, and even partial amnesia has become so well known among rape victims and survivors of natural disasters (Herman 1992; Madakasira and O'Brian 1987; Spiegel 1990; Wilkinson 1983) that these symptoms have been incorporated as DSM-IV diagnostic criteria for posttraumatic stress disorder (American Psychiatric Association 1994, pp. 424–429) and acute stress disorder (pp. 429–432).

Even more recently, investigators (Coons 1992; Coons and Milstein 1992; Coons et al. 1988; Putnam et al. 1986; Ross et al. 1989) have found that the amnesia characteristic of most of the dissociative disorders is linked to childhood trauma. The incidence of childhood trauma in dissociative identity disorder (DID) (formerly multiple personality disorder) varies from 85% to 98%, and the incidence of amnesia is virtually 100% (Coons et al. 1988; Putnam et al. 1986; Ross et al. 1989). In the studies involving DID, it is unclear whether the memories are merely dissociated into another personality state and available just to that personality state or whether the memories are totally forgotten or repressed and unavailable to any personality state. Of course, both mechanisms may be at work.

Studies Involving Predominantly Sexual Trauma

The most recent literature on recovered memories primarily involves memories of childhood sexual abuse. With one exception, all of these studies have been published since 1993 (Table 10–2).

Herman and Schatzow (1987) studied 53 female outpatients who had participated in short-term group psychotherapy for incest survivors and found that 74% of the patients had been able to corroborate their abuse experiences from perpetrator admissions, observations of other family members, physical evidence, or the discovery that another sibling had also been sexually abused. Onset of abuse ranged from ages 2 to 19 years, with an average age of 8. Abuse that began in or continued

Table 10–2.   Studies involving amnesia associated primarily with sexual trauma

Study	Nature of population	Number in series	Percent with amnesia (full or partial)	Confirmation of trauma
Herman and Schatzow (1987)	Female incest victims	53	64	74%
Briere and Conte (1993)	Adult psychiatric patients (mostly female)	450	59	No
Albach (1993)	Women reporting childhood incest	97	88	No
Binder et al. (1994)	Women with childhood sexual abuse	30	43	No
Burgess (1994)	Female military dependents sexually abused in day care	19	42	100%
Cameron (1994)	Women with childhood sexual abuse	60	65	No
Roesler and Wind (1994)	Female incest victims	228	28	No
Loftus et al. (1994)	Women with childhood sexual abuse	57	31	No
Feldman-Summers and Pope (1994)	Psychologists	79	40	46%
Williams (1994, 1995)	Women with childhood sexual abuse	129	48	100%
Elliott and Briere (1995)	Victims of childhood sexual abuse (55% female)	505	42	No
van der Kolk and Fisler (1995)	Men and women with childhood trauma (primarily sexual abuse)	36	42	75%
Tromp et al. (1995)	Employed women	1,037	—	No

into adolescence was never completely forgotten, and the most severe memory deficits were associated with either violent/sadistic abuse or abuse that began in early childhood and ended before adolescence.

Briere and Conte (1993) studied 450 adult psychiatric patients who reported sexual abuse histories and found that 59% had experienced amnesia for the abuse at some point in their lives before age 18. Predictors of amnesia included earlier age at onset of sexual abuse, longer abuse duration, larger number of abusers, greater current psychiatric symptomatology, and more violent abuse. Interestingly, guilt or shame was found not to be related to amnesia. No attempt was made to verify abuse histories in this study.

Albach (1993) studied 97 women who reported childhood incest and compared them with 65 female control subjects, matched for age and educational level, who denied childhood incest. The control subjects were asked to describe memories of other unpleasant childhood events. Of the women who were sexually abused, the duration was longer than 1 year in 90%. Violence was used in 43%. The mean duration of sexual abuse was 15 years. Amnesia was not correlated to age at onset of abuse, duration or frequency of abuse, or use of violence. Triggers for memory recovery included discovering that their own daughters had been abused, personal revictimization, illness or death of the perpetrator, and sensory cues (tactile, olfactory, visual, or auditory). Significantly more sexually abused subjects had either complete (29%) or partial amnesia (59%) for the abuse than the control group had for their experiences of unpleasant events.

Binder et al. (1994) studied 30 women who had been sexually abused as children and found that 43% had some amnesia for the abuse. In contrast to Briere and Conte's (1993) study, they found no relation in age at onset of abuse, length of abuse, number of abusers, and violence between their amnesic and nonamnesic samples. They did not attempt to independently verify sexual abuse histories. Interestingly, eight patients' conditions were described in detail, including how their memories were recovered. In three of these patients, memories were recovered through questionable memory enhancement techniques such as hypnosis ($n = 2$) and dreaming ($n = 1$). Burgess (1994, reported in Whitfield 1995, p. 72) followed up 19 military-dependent children with sexual abuse corroborated by day-care-center staff. At 10-year follow-up, 42% had either partially or completely forgotten the trauma. The abuse had occurred at a mean age of 2.5 years. Cameron (1994) interviewed and followed up, during a 6-year period, 60 women who had been sexually abused in childhood; 23% had partially forgotten and 42% had completely forgotten that they were sexually abused in childhood.

Roesler and Wind (1994) studied 228 adult women who reported incestuous experiences before age 18. The mean age at onset of abuse was 6.0 years, and the mean duration of abuse was 7.6 years. Twenty-eight percent had repressed memories of their abuse. The investigators did not seek to independently verify abuse histories in this study.

Loftus et al. (1994) studied 105 women in outpatient therapy for substance abuse, 54% of whom reported childhood sexual abuse. Of the sexually abused patients, 19% had completely forgotten and 12% had partially forgotten the abuse. The forgetting of abuse was not related to the number of abusers, frequency of abuse, or violent nature of the abuse, but it was associated with more intense feelings at the time of the abuse. As in most of the other studies, the investigators did not attempt to independently verify that the abuse had occurred.

Feldman-Summers and Pope (1994) administered a questionnaire to a national sample of psychologists. Of the respondents, 79 (24%) reported childhood abuse, 40% of whom had once been unable to remember the abuse. Those who reported being abused by more than one person were more likely to have amnesia than those who reported only one abuser, but amnesia was not correlated with severity of abuse. Both physical and sexual abuse were subject to periods of forgetting. Triggers for remembering abuse included reading a book or watching television or a movie (25.0%), being reminded about the abuse by an observer of the abuse (18.8%), engaging in psychotherapy (56.2%) or a self-help group (6.2%), and having an experience such as caring for others who were abused or making love (28.1%); no particular triggers for remembering abuse were found in 9.4% of the sample. Half of those who reported amnesia indicated that they had corroboration of the abuse. These types of corroboration included acknowledgment by the abuser (15.6%), acknowledgment by an observer (21.9%), notation in a diary by the victim (6.2%), reports of someone else being abused by the same perpetrator (15.6%), and evidence from medical records (6.2%).

Elliott and Briere (1995) studied 505 individuals (55% female) who had been sexually abused; 42% described full or partial amnesia for the experience. Delayed recall of the abuse was associated with the use of threats by the perpetrator at the time of the abuse and their perception of the abuse as very distressing. Factors not related to recall included age at the time of abuse, frequency of abuse, duration of abuse, use of actual physical force, and presence of sexual penetration.

Two recent studies provide data that traumatic memories are different from other types of memory. van der Kolk and Fisler (1995) studied 46 subjects (36 women and 10 men) with posttraumatic stress disorder who had endured a variety of traumas in both childhood and adulthood. However, the majority of the traumas (55%) consisted of childhood sexual abuse or assault. Of the 36 subjects with childhood trauma, 42% had either partial or total amnesia for the trauma, and 75% reported confirmation of the trauma through family members or court or hospital records. The initial return of their memories consisted of sensory (visual, olfactory, auditory, and kinesthetic) and affective experiences that emerged prior to a coherent narrative. Tromp et al. (1995) studied memories among 1,037 employed women and found that memories of rape experiences were less clear and vivid, less well remembered, and less talked about than other types of memories, both pleasant and unpleasant.

In the most sophisticated studies to date, Williams (1994, 1995) obtained follow-up data on 129 of 206 women who had documented evidence from a hospital emergency department for childhood sexual assault. Thirty-eight percent had no memory of the incident of sexual assault, and an additional 10% had forgotten the assault at one time but had subsequently remembered it. Amnesia was not associated with violence or repeated abuse; however, it was correlated with younger age at onset of the abuse and abuse by someone familiar. In the five case histories described in detail in the second paper (1995), it appears that memories of sexual assault were not immediately forgotten. These women stated that they began forgetting anywhere from 2 to 16 years after the assault and did not begin remembering the assault until their early 20s.

Although not related to recovered memories, Terr's studies (1988, 1991) of 20 children who had documented trauma prior to age 5 are instructive. These children were interviewed about the trauma an average of 4.4 years after it had occurred. She found that verbal recall of trauma was rare before age 36 months but that behavioral memories consisting of precise reenactments of the trauma were virtually universal and accurately conveyed the details of the trauma. Also, single episodes of trauma were more easily remembered than multiple episodes, and traumas of short duration were more easily remembered than traumas of long duration. Terr established that before age 28–36 months, full verbal memories of traumas did not occur.

Only two studies have confirmed trauma, consisting primarily of childhood physical and sexual abuse, in patients with DID and dissociative disorder not otherwise specified. In the first (Coons and Milstein 1986), 85% of 20 patients with DID had histories of childhood abuse, which were verified by either family members or emergency room reports. In the second study (Coons 1994a), a retrospective chart review of 19 cases of child and adolescent DID and dissociative disorder not otherwise specified, 8 of 9 patients with DID and 9 of 10 patients with dissociative disorder not otherwise specified had child abuse, which was verified by various family members and by medical, psychiatric, and police reports.

In contrast to the considerable confirmation of childhood physical and sexual abuse memories in the Feldman-Summers and Pope (1994) and Herman and Schatzow (1987) studies, reports of satanic ritual abuse have not received significant confirmation. These reports of multigenerational abuse include bizarre rituals of torture, perverted sex, human and animal sacrifice, cannibalism, and the breeding of babies for human sacrifice. Four studies of subjects reporting such practices (Bottoms et al. 1996; Coons 1994b; J. S. LaFontaine, "The extent and nature of organized and ritual abuse: a report to the department of health," unpublished manuscript, London, 1994; Weir and Wheatcroft 1995) found no corroboration of such horrific practices, and law enforcement agencies have not been able to find corroboration (Lanning 1992). However, evidence has been found that some individuals, usually acting alone, use paraphernalia, such as altars and candles, during their ritualistic abuse of children.

Present Study

Purpose

The purpose of the present study was to assess whether memories of reported trauma had been forgotten in patients with dissociative disorders and, if so, how the memories returned. The experiences of forgetting and remembering in patients with dissociative disorders were compared with the experiences of a control group of subjects with affective disorders but not dissociative disorders.

Methods

Subjects

The subjects were 50 consecutive patients in whom we (P. M. C. and E. S. B.) diagnosed dissociative disorders based on DSM-IV criteria. These patients included 28 with DID (3 were in remission), 20 with dissociative disorder not otherwise specified, and 1 each with dissociative amnesia and dissociative fugue. The control group consisted of 25 consecutive patients with various DSM-IV affective disorders, including 11 with major depression; 4 with schizoaffective disorder (depressed, in remission); 3 each with dysthymia, adjustment disorder with depression, and depression not otherwise specified; and 1 with organic affective disorder (depressed) secondary to hypothyroidism.

Of the 50 dissociative disorder patients, 46 (92%) were women and 48 (96%) were white. Mean age was 34.9 years (range, 16–63 years). Marital status was 23 (46%) single, 11 (22%) married, and 16 (32%) separated or divorced. Mean educational level was 13.8 years. Occupations included 14 (28%) professional or managerial, 7 (14%) skilled or semiskilled, 2 (4%) unskilled, 14 (28%) disabled or unemployed, 6 (12%) homemakers, 6 (12%) students, and 1 (2%) retired. Religious affiliation was predominantly Protestant (52%), with 7 (14%) Catholic, 2 (4%) Jewish, and 15 (30%) who professed no religious affiliation.

Of the 25 affective disorder patients, 20 (80%) were women; all except 1 patient were white. Mean age was 33.2 years (range, 19–59 years). Marital status was 12 (48%) single, 8 (32%) married, and 5 (20%) separated or divorced. Mean educational level was 15.3 years. Occupations included 12 (48%) professional or managerial, 6 (24%) skilled or semi-skilled, 3 (12%) unemployed or disabled, 2 (8%) homemakers, and 2 (8%) students. Religious affiliation was primarily Protestant (80%), with 1 (4%) Catholic and 4 (16%) who professed no religious affiliation.

Procedures

During their psychiatric examination, outpatients were given a trauma questionnaire to assess demographic data, types of trauma experienced both in childhood and in adulthood, whether the trauma was forgotten, circumstances under which the memory returned (fully awake, flashbacks, dreams, hypnosis, guided imagery, or relaxation), triggers for memory return, and the therapist's attitude toward memories. Statistical comparison between the dissociative disorder and affective disorder groups was calculated with a Yates-corrected χ^2.

Results

No significant differences in age, sex, race, marital status, or religious affiliation were found between the dissociative disorder and affective disorder groups. However, significantly more patients in the affective disorder group (12%) compared with the dissociative disorder group (4%) had 20 or more years of education ($\chi^2 = 7.150$, df $= 1$, $P = .006$). In addition, the number of subjects in the dissociative disorder group (24%) compared with the affective disorder group (4%) who were disabled tended toward significance ($\chi^2 = 3.362$, df $= 1$, $P = .067$).

Traumatic Experiences

A greater incidence of all types of child abuse (i.e., physical, sexual, or verbal abuse; abandonment; and neglect), rape in adulthood, and spouse abuse was reported by the dissociative disorder group. In the dissociative disorder and affective disorder groups, 96% and 56%, respectively, reported the incidence of any type of childhood abuse (see Table 10–3).

Only 17 (34%) of the dissociative disorder patients and 4 (16%) of the affective disorder patients had ever discussed their child abuse experiences directly with their abuser. None had ever filed a lawsuit against their abusers. Interestingly, half of the dissociative disorder group felt that their therapist believed fully or partially all of their traumatic experiences, whereas the other half felt that their therapists were neutral and encouraged them to discover for themselves whether the reported traumatic experiences did, in fact, happen.

Table 10–3. Experiences of trauma in patients with dissociative and affective disorders

Type of trauma	Dissociative disorder group (N = 50) n (%)	Affective disorder group (N = 25) n (%)	P value[a]
Child abuse			
Physical	39 (78)	5 (20)	<.001
Sexual	42 (84)	5 (20)	<.001
Verbal	41 (82)	5 (20)	<.001
Neglect	26 (52)	2 (8)	<.001
Abandonment	23 (46)	3 (12)	.008
None	2 (4)	11 (44)	<.001
Natural disaster			
Tornado	9 (18)	2 (8)	ID
Flood	3 (6)	0	ID
Earthquake	4 (8)	0	NS
Hurricane	4 (8)	3 (12)	NS
Fire	10 (20)	1 (4)	ID
Other			
Accident	13 (26)	2 (8)	NS
Rape	24 (48)	4 (16)	.014
Spouse abuse	20 (40)	3 (12)	.027

Note. ID = insufficient data; NS = not significant (*P* > .05).
[a]df = 1 for all values.

Memory Return

Loss of memory for trauma. In the dissociative disorder group, 96% of subjects reported that they had forgotten, either partially or fully, various forms of trauma compared with only 24% of the control group. Of the patients in the dissociative disorder group, 56%–86% forgot, either partially or fully, their childhood abuse experiences; 25%–66% forgot natural disasters; and 30%–45% forgot other types of trauma, including rape, accidents, and spouse abuse. Although the patients in the affective disorder group reported forgetting traumatic experiences at a much lower rate, they reported forgetting instances of verbal and sexual abuse, rape, and tornadoes. Although dissociative disorder patients reported higher instances of trauma in most cases, insufficient data from the affective disorder group prevented statistical comparisons for most types of trauma between the two groups. Of the three types of trauma for which the data were sufficient, only the difference in forgetting physical abuse was statistically significant (see Table 10–4).

Table 10–4.   Loss of memory (either full or partial) for trauma

Type of trauma	Dissociative disorder group ($N = 50$) n	Affective disorder group ($N = 25$) n	P value[a]
Child abuse			
Physical	28	0	.008
Sexual	36	3	ID
Verbal	24	1	ID
Neglect	17	0	NS
Abandonment	17	0	NS
Natural disaster			
Tornado	4	2	ID
Flood	2	0	ID
Earthquake	1	0	ID
Hurricane	2	0	ID
Fire	4	0	ID
Other			
Accident	4	0	ID
Rape	11	2	ID
Spouse abuse	6	0	ID

Note.   ID = insufficient data; NS = not significant ($P > .05$).
[a]df = 1 for all values.

Method of memory return.   Most instances of memory return in affective disorder patients occurred when they were fully awake. In contrast, among the dissociative disorder patients, memories returned in a variety of both awake and altered states of consciousness. In many instances, their memories returned in the form of flashbacks. Many memories returned in the form of dreams, while under hypnosis, during twilight states, or during therapeutic relaxation or guided imagery (see Table 10–5).

Triggers for memory return.   Return of memories in both groups was triggered by a wide variety of experiences including visual and auditory stimuli, retraumatization, hearing about someone else's trauma, reading, or group therapy sessions (Table 10–6). While the dissociative disorder patients were in treatment, their memories were as likely to return outside of the therapeutic situation as within. In half of the dissociative disorder patients, memories returned prior to the initiation of their treatment.

Table 10–5.   Method of memory return

Method of return	Dissociative disorder group (N = 48) n (%)	Affective disorder group (N = 6) n (%)	P value[a]
Flashbacks	38 (79)	0	<.001
Awake	36 (75)	5 (83)	NS
Dreams	24 (50)	2 (33)	NS
Twilight states	19 (40)	0	NS
Relaxation	13 (27)	0	NS
Guided imagery	7 (15)	0	NS
Hypnosis	10 (21)	0	NS

Note.   NS = not significant (P > .05).
[a]df = 1.

Table 10–6.   Triggers for memory return

Triggers	Dissociative disorder group (N = 48) n (%)	Affective disorder group (N = 6) n (%)	P value[a]
Visual stimuli	34 (71)	4 (67)	ID
Auditory stimuli	27 (56)	2 (33)	ID
Another trauma	23 (48)	1 (17)	ID
Someone else's trauma	18 (38)	4 (67)	ID
Reading	17 (35)	3 (50)	ID
Group therapy	10 (21)	2 (33)	ID
No particular trigger	6 (13)	0	NS

Note.   ID = insufficient data; NS = not significant (P > .05).
[a]df = 1 for all values.

Discussion and Conclusion

Summary of Studies of Traumatic Memory

To summarize the studies on traumatic memory to date, it is clear that memories of trauma can be partially or completely forgotten by 18%–59% of victims. Traumatic memories can be repressed for all types of trauma, including physical and sexual childhood abuse, rape, concentration camp or hostage experiences, combat, and natural disasters, but memory loss for childhood abuse appears to be the most common. Complete loss of memories of trauma usually occurs when the trauma takes place before adolescence. Amnesia for trauma is correlated with earlier onset of trauma and multiple types of trauma. In most of the studies reviewed, the trauma occurred after the usual period of infantile amnesia (birth to age 2.5–3 years). Traumatic memories may not be immediately forgotten. Repression may occur several years after the trauma has occurred. Repressed memories of child abuse can be corroborated in 50%–75% of cases. It is becoming more clear that traumatic memory is quite different from other forms of memory.

Amnesia for traumatic events can occur in several psychiatric illnesses. Amnesia is a diagnostic criterion for posttraumatic stress disorder, acute stress disorder, dissociative amnesia and fugue, and DID.

Traumatic events that occurred during childhood may not be remembered until the late teens and, most often, not until the third and fourth decades of life. The return of traumatic memories can be triggered by many events, including visual and auditory stimuli, hearing or reading about someone else's trauma, retraumatization, and group or individual psychotherapy.

Pseudomemories of traumatic events can definitely occur. Examples of pseudomemories include memories of infancy, many satanic ritual abuse reports, past-life experiences, and UFO abductions. The use of hypnosis, suggestive interview techniques, dream analysis, guided imagery, and fantasy predispose toward pseudomemory formation.

The existence of verbal childhood memories before age 1 year is impossible, and the veracity of verbal memories between ages 1 and 2 years should be highly suspect. The veracity of satanic ritual abuse memories is highly suspect. The reliability of adult memories of childhood abuse beginning before age 2 years is also highly suspect. At present, outside corroboration is the only way to determine whether a particular memory is reliable.

Comparison of Results With Those of Previous Studies

Our study confirmed and extended the results of previous studies on the forgetting of traumatic memories. We found that traumatic memories can be forgotten for childhood abuse, natural disasters, rape, and spouse abuse. We confirmed that there are many different types of triggers for traumatic memory return, including visual and auditory stimuli, retraumatization, hearing or reading about someone else's trauma, and group psychotherapy. Trauma occurs more often in DID and dissociative disorder not otherwise specified than in affective disorders. Forgetting of trauma appears to occur more in those with dissociative disorders than in those with affective disorders.

In dissociative disorder patients, we found that memories could return in the context of highly questionable therapeutic practices for memory retrieval, including dream analysis, hypnosis, and guided imagery. However, the return of traumatic memories was not necessarily related to therapy but could occur during relaxation or twilight states outside of therapy.

Limitations of This Study

One of the difficulties with our study was the small sample size, especially of the affective disorder patients. We were not always able to make statistical comparisons between the dissociative disorder and affective disorder groups. In future studies, investigators who want to compare the differences in traumatic forgetting between those with dissociative disorder and other diagnostic groups must use larger sample sizes (very much larger if items with low frequency of reporting are included). In this study, we did not confirm that the traumatic events had actually taken place. This and most of the other studies were self-reports of memory loss and later recovery, which might not be accurate. However, some of the previously cited studies on traumatic forgetting found considerable confirmation of trauma, lending some credibility to reports of trauma among psychiatric outpatients. In addition, in past studies on dissociative disorder, confirmation of trauma has been very high (Coons 1994a; Coons and Milstein 1986).

Treatment Recommendations

At present, clinicians should follow published treatment guidelines for patients with recovered memories of trauma. The following is our advice to clinicians who treat dissociative disorders:

Use psychodynamic psychotherapy.   Although medication is often useful in the treatment of dissociative disorders and comorbid post-traumatic stress disorder (Davidson 1992; Loewenstein 1991), psychodynamic psychotherapy should be the primary mode of treatment for most of these patients (Kluft 1995). To avoid a worsening of the patient's symptomatology, the clinician should be careful to respect the patient's dissociative defenses by ensuring safety, proceeding slowly, and not overusing abreaction (Kluft 1995; Segall 1995). In addition, to avoid regression, clinicians should not utilize fringe therapies such as exorcism (Bowman 1993) or reparenting (Greaves 1988).

Maintain therapeutic neutrality.   If patients ask whether the clinician believes that they were abused, the clinician should respond that abuse is possible, but the clinician cannot confirm that the abuse occurred because he or she was not an observer. It is important to explore why patients focus on belief. Were they not believed as children? Do they have a problem with trust? Lawsuits against abusers should not be encouraged, and, if a lawsuit is filed, the clinician should not involve himself or herself in a dual relationship by being both the patient's therapist and expert witness.

Educate both yourself and your patient about memory and enhancement procedures.   The clinician should obtain collateral information to assess accuracy of memory. Hypnosis and Amytal sodium should be used rarely for memory retrieval. However, if either technique is used, the clinician should obtain informed consent and should adhere to guidelines for treatment (American Society of Clinical Hypnosis 1995) or use in forensic contexts (American Medical Association 1985). Suggestive interview techniques in memory retrieval should not be used. Suggestive questions should be avoided if hypnosis is utilized. The use of guided imagery or dream analysis for memory retrieval should be avoided altogether.

Stay within the limits of your clinical competence.   If the clinician is not trained in psychodynamic therapy, the patient should be referred to someone well trained in this therapy. Consultations should be obtained when the clinician is treating difficult patients. If the clinician contemplates using hypnosis, he or she should have received proper training in its use from an accredited organization.

Maintain good records.   The clinician should document the symptoms and memories with which patients initially present, the use of informed consent, the gathering of collateral information, whether memories are retrieved inside or outside of treatment, the triggers for memories, and any methods used to retrieve memories. The clinician should adequately document that he or she followed current guidelines for the treatment of DID (International Society for the Study of Dissociation 1994) and the use of memory enhancement procedures to aid in defending against malpractice lawsuits regarding false memories.

A Possible Biological Basis for Traumatic Forgetting

Recently, Bremner et al. (1995a) reviewed the neuroanatomical correlates of the effects of stress on memory. It has previously been shown that the limbic regions of the brain mediate memory function, fear-related behaviors, and the stress response. More specifically, recent research has shown that the hippocampal volume of patients with posttraumatic stress disorder is decreased as compared with those without posttraumatic stress disorder (Bremner et al. 1995b). The constant outpouring of glucocorticosteroids that occurs with chronic stress or trauma may somehow damage the hippocampus. If this is so, a mechanism may exist to explain not only why traumatic memories may be forgotten but also why they may not be remembered correctly.

Directions for Future Research

Many questions remain about traumatic memory. How and why are memories forgotten? Are shame or guilt involved in forgetting? Is damage to the hippocampus involved in patients with dissociative disorders and in others who have been traumatized and forgotten their trauma? Does damage to the hippocampus affect the accuracy of remembering in those who have been traumatized? Does the use of secrecy or threats by the perpetrators of child abuse affect whether the abuse is forgotten? Are clinical methods available to distinguish accurate from inaccurate memories? For those therapeutic techniques believed to distort accurate recall, how severely are memories distorted for each of these? For example, are memories retrieved from dreams ever accurate, or are most memories derived from flashbacks accurate? Most of all, as Janet implied in 1925, rules for discerning the accuracy of traumatic memories and for proper treatment are urgently needed. The answers to these and other questions await further research in this significant area.

References

Albach F: Freud's Verleidingstheorie: Incest, Trauma, and Hysterie [Freud's Seduction Hypothesis: Incest, Trauma, and Hysteria]. Amsterdam, Academisch Proefschrift, de Universiteit van Amsterdam, 1993

Allen JG: The spectrum of accuracy in memories of childhood trauma. Harvard Review of Psychiatry 3:84–95, 1995

American Medical Association, Council on Scientific Affairs: The status of refreshing recollection by the use of hypnosis. JAMA 253:1918–1923, 1985

American Medical Association, Council on Scientific Affairs: Report 5-A-94: Memories of Childhood Abuse. Chicago, IL, American Medical Association, 1994

American Psychiatric Association: Diagnostic and Statistical Manual of Mental Disorders, 4th Edition. Washington, DC, American Psychiatric Association, 1994

American Psychiatric Association, Board of Trustees: Statement on memories of sexual abuse. Int J Clin Exp Hypn 42:261–264, 1994

American Society of Clinical Hypnosis: Clinical Hypnosis and Memory: Guidelines for Clinicians and for Forensic Hypnosis. Chicago, IL, American Society of Clinical Hypnosis, 1995

Applied Cognitive Psychology 8:281–435, 1994

Archibald HC, Tuddenham RD: Persistent stress reaction after combat. Arch Gen Psychiatry 12:475–481, 1956

Binder RL, McNiel DE, Goldstone RL: Patterns of recall of childhood sexual abuse as described by adult survivors. Bull Am Acad Psychiatry Law 22:357–366, 1994

Bloom P: Clinical guidelines in using hypnosis in uncovering memories of sexual abuse: a master class commentary. Int J Clin Exp Hypn 42:173–178, 1994

Bottoms BL, Goodman GS, Shauer PR: An analysis of ritualistic and religion-related child abuse allegations. Law and Human Behavior 20:1–34, 1996

Bowman ES: Clinical and spiritual effects of exorcism in fifteen patients with multiple personality disorder. Dissociation 6:222–238, 1993

Bremner JD, Krystal JH, Southwick SM, et al: Functional neuroanatomical correlates of the effects of stress on memory. J Trauma Stress 8:527–553, 1995a

Bremner JD, Randall P, Scott TM, et al: MRI-based measurement of hippocampal volume in combat-related posttraumatic stress disorder. Am J Psychiatry 152:973–981, 1995b

Briere J, Conte J: Self-reported amnesia in adults molested as children. J Trauma Stress 6:21–31, 1993

British Psychological Society: Recovered memories. Psychologist 8:507–508, 1995

Cameron C: Women survivors confronting their abusers: issues, decisions, and outcomes. Journal of Child Sexual Abuse 3:7–35, 1994

Ceci SJ, Bruck M: Suggestibility of the child witness: a historical review and synthesis. Psychol Bull 113:413–439, 1993

Consciousness Cognition 3(3–4):265–469, 1994

Consciousness Cognition 4(1):63–134, 1995

Coons PM: Dissociative disorder not otherwise specified: a clinical investigation of 50 cases with suggestions for treatment. Dissociation 5:187–195, 1992

Coons PM: Confirmation of childhood abuse in child and adolescent cases of multiple personality disorder and dissociative disorder not otherwise specified. J Nerv Ment Dis 182:461–464, 1994a

Coons PM: Reports of satanic ritual abuse: further implications of pseudomemories. Percept Mot Skills 78:1376–1378, 1994b

Coons PM, Milstein V: Psychosexual differences in multiple personality: characteristics, etiology, and treatment. J Clin Psychiatry 47:106–110, 1986

Coons PM, Milstein V: Psychogenic amnesia: a clinical investigation of 25 cases. Dissociation 5:73–79, 1992

Coons PM, Bowman ES, Milstein V: Multiple personality disorder: a clinical investigation of 50 cases. J Nerv Ment Dis 176:519–527, 1988

Counseling Psychologist 23(2):181–363, 1995

Cronin JA: Science and the admissibility of evidence: the latest FMSF tactics. Treating Abuse Today 5(1):30–37, 1995

Davidson J: Drug therapy of post-traumatic stress disorder. Br J Psychiatry 160:309–314, 1992

Elliott DM, Briere J: Posttraumatic stress associated with delayed recall of sexual abuse: a general population study. J Trauma Stress 8:629–647, 1995

Feldman-Summers S, Pope KS: The experience of forgetting childhood abuse: a national survey of psychologists. J Consult Clin Psychol 62:636–639, 1994

Fisher C: Amnesic states in war neuroses: the psychogenesis of fugues. Psychoanal Q 14:437–458, 1944

Fowler C: A pragmatic approach to early childhood memories: shifting the focus from truth to clinical utility. Psychotherapy 31:676–686, 1994

Frankel FH: The concept of flashbacks in historical perspective. Int J Clin Exp Hypn 42:321–336, 1994

Goldfield AE, Mollica RF, Pesanvento BH: The psychical and psychological sequelae of torture: symptomatology and diagnosis. JAMA 25:2725–2729, 1988

Golston JC: A false memory syndrome conference: activist accused and their professional allies talk about science, law, and family reconciliation. Treating Abuse Today 5(1):24–30, 1995

Greaves GB: Common errors in the treatment of multiple personality disorder. Dissociation 1:61–66, 1988

Gutheil TG: True or false memories of sexual abuse? A forensic psychiatric view. Psychiatric Annals 23:527–531, 1993

Hammond DC: Clinical hypnosis and memory: guidelines for clinicians. Newsletter of the International Society for the Study of Dissociation 13(4):1,9, 1995

Henderson JL, Moore M: The psychoneuroses of war. N Engl J Med 230:274–278, 1944

Hendin H, Hags AP, Singer P: The reliving experience in Vietnam veterans with posttraumatic stress disorder. Compr Psychiatry 23:163–173, 1984

Herman JL: Trauma and Recovery. New York, Basic Books, 1992

Herman JL, Schatzow E: Recovery and verification of memories of childhood sexual trauma. Psychoanalytic Psychology 4:1–14, 1987

Int J Clin Exp Hypn 42(4):258–455, 1994

Int J Clin Exp Hypn 43(2):109–248, 1995

International Society for the Study of Dissociation: ISSD Guidelines for Treating Dissociative Identity Disorder (Multiple Personality Disorder) in Adults. Skokie, IL, International Society for the Study of Dissociation, 1994

Jaffe R: Dissociative phenomena in former concentration camp inmates. Int J Psychoanal 49:310–312, 1968

Janet P: Psychological Healing: A Historical and Clinical Study, Vol 1. New York, Macmillan, 1925, p 670

Journal of Psychohistory 23(2):119–190, 1995

J Trauma Stress 8(4):501–726, 1995

Kalman G: On combat-neurosis. Int J Soc Psychiatry 23:195–203, 1977

Kihlstrom JF: The trauma-memory argument. Consciousness Cognition 4:63–67, 1995

Kinzie JD: Posttraumatic effects and their treatment among Southeast Asia refugees, in International Handbook of Traumatic Stress Syndromes. Edited by Wilson JP, Raphael B. New York, Plenum, 1993, pp 311–319

Kluft RP: Dissociative identity disorder, part II: treatment. Directions in Psychiatry 15(24):1–7, 1995

Lanning KV: A law enforcement perspective on allegations of ritual abuse, in Out of Darkness: Exploring Satanism and Ritual Abuse. Edited by Sakheim DK, Levine SE. New York, Lexington Books, 1992, pp 109–144

Lindsay DS, Read JD: Psychotherapy and memories of childhood sexual abuse: a cognitive perspective. Applied Cognitive Psychology 8:281–338, 1994

Loewenstein RJ: Rational psychopharmacotherapy in the treatment of multiple personality disorder. Psychiatr Clin North Am 14:721–740, 1991

Loftus EF: The reality of repressed memories. Am Psychol 48:517–537, 1993

Loftus EF, Polonsky S, Fullilove MT: Memories of childhood sexual abuse: remembering and repressing. Psychology of Women Quarterly 18:67–84, 1994

Lynn SJ, Nash MR: Truth in memory: ramifications for psychotherapy and hypnotherapy. Am J Clin Hypn 36:194–208, 1994

Madakasira S, O'Brian K: Acute posttraumatic stress disorder in victims of natural disaster. J Nerv Ment Dis 175:286–290, 1987

McHugh PR, Butterfield MI: Do patients' recovered memories of sexual abuse constitute a "false memory syndrome"? Psychiatric News 28(23):18, 1993

Modai I: Forgetting childhood: a defense mechanism against psychosis in a holocaust survivor. Clinical Gerontologist 14(3):61–67, 1994

Niederland WG: Clinical observations on the "survivor syndrome." Int J Psychoanal 49:313–315, 1968

Orne MT, Whitehouse WC, Dinges DF, et al: Reconstructing memory through hypnosis: forensic and clinical implications, in Hypnosis and Memory. Edited by Pettinati HM. New York, Guilford, 1988, pp 21–63

Pope HG, Hudson JL: Can memories of childhood sexual abuse be repressed? Psychol Med 25:121–126, 1995

Powell RA, Boer DP: Did Freud mislead patients to confabulate memories of abuse? Psychol Rep 74:1283–1298, 1995

Psychiatric Annals 25(12):713–735, 1995

Putnam FW, Guroff JJ, Silberman EK, et al: The clinical phenomenology of multiple personality disorder: a review of 100 recent cases. J Clin Psychiatry 47:285–293, 1986

Roesler TA, Wind TW: Telling the secret: adult women describe their disclosures of incest. Journal of Interpersonal Violence 9:327–338, 1994

Ross CA, Norton G, Wozney K: Multiple personality disorder: an analysis of 236 cases. Can J Psychiatry 34:413–418, 1989

Sargant W, Slater E: Amnesic syndromes of war. Proceedings of the Royal Society of Medicine 34:757–764, 1941

Segall SR: Misalliances and misadventures in the treatment of dissociative disorders, in Dissociative Identity Disorder: Theoretical and Treatment Controversies. Edited by Cohen LM, Berzoff JN, Elin MR. Northvale, NJ, Jason Aronson, 1995, pp 379–412

Sonneberg SM, Blank AS, Talbott JA: The Traumas of War: Stress and Recovery in Vietnam Veterans. Washington, DC, American Psychiatric Press, 1985

Spanos NP, Burgess CA, Burgess MF: Past-life identities, UFO abductions, and satanic ritual abuse: a social construction of memories. Int J Clin Exp Hypn 42:433–446, 1994

Spence DP: Narrative truth and putative child abuse. Int J Clin Exp Hypn 42:289–303, 1995

Spiegel D: Trauma, dissociation, and hypnosis, in Incest-Related Syndromes of Adult Psychopathology. Edited by Kluft RP. Washington, DC, American Psychiatric Press, 1990, pp 247–261

Terr L: What happens to early memories of old trauma? A study of twenty children under age five at the time of documented traumatic events. J Am Acad Child Adolesc Psychiatry 27:96–104, 1988

Terr L: Childhood traumas: an outline and overview. Am J Psychiatry 148:10–20, 1991

Thom DA, Fenton N: Amnesias in war cases. American Journal of Insanity 7:437–448, 1920

Torrie A: Psychosomatic casualties in the Middle East. Lancet 1:139–143, 1944

Tromp S, Koss MP, Figuredo AJ, et al: Are rape memories different: a comparison of rape, other unpleasant, and pleasant memories among employed women. J Trauma Stress 8:607–627, 1995

Usher JA, Neisser U: Childhood amnesia in the beginnings of memory for four early life events. J Exp Psychol Gen 2:155–165, 1993

van der Hart O, Nijenhuis E: Amnesia for traumatic experiences. Hypnos 22:73–86, 1995

van der Kolk BA, Fisler R: Dissociation and the fragmentary nature of traumatic memories: overview and exploratory study. J Trauma Stress 8:505–525, 1995

Wakefield H, Underwager R: Uncovering memories of alleged sexual abuse: the therapists who do it. Issues in Child Abuse Accusations 4:197–213, 1992

Wakefield H, Underwager R: Return of the Furies: An Investigation Into Recovered Memory Therapy. Chicago, IL, Open Court, 1994

Watkins JG: Dealing with the problem of "false memory" in clinic and court. Journal of Psychiatry and the Law 21:297–317, 1993

Weir IK, Wheatcroft MS: Allegations of children's involvement in ritual sexual abuse: clinical experience in 20 cases. Child Abuse Negl 19:491–505, 1995

Whitfield CL: Memory and Abuse: Remembering and Healing the Effects of Trauma. Dearfield Beach, FL, Heath Communications, 1995

Wilkinson CB: Aftermath of a disaster: collapse of the Hyatt Regency Hotel skywalks. Am J Psychiatry 140:1134–1139, 1983

Williams LM: Recall of childhood trauma: a prospective study of women's memories of child sexual abuse. J Consult Clin Psychol 62:1167–1176, 1994

Williams LM: Recovered memories of abuse in women with documented child sexual victimization histories. J Trauma Stress 8:649–673, 1995

Yapko MD: Suggestions of Abuse: True and False Memories of Childhood Sexual Traumas. New York, Simon & Schuster, 1994

Afterword to Section II

David Spiegel, M.D., Section Editor

In the chapters in Section II, a sizable body of research and systematic clinical observation is reviewed. Despite disparate professional interests and orientations, common ground is found. The authors generally agree that memory of any event is a reconstructive process, a matching of schema with memory trace, subject to suggestive influence and the need for affect regulation. At the same time, memory defects, including traumatic amnesia, are observed commonly after traumatic stressors, consistent with the alteration in cognitive function that commonly occurs during trauma. The evidence that suggestion can alter memory retrieval does not prove that memory, even recovered memory, is inherently unreliable. Rather, it provides further evidence that memory of real traumatic events can be repressed with suggestion, just as false memories can be suggested. Indeed, some research indicates that people vulnerable to suggestion effects are more likely to have real memories of events similar to those suggested: the schema exists even though the event did not.

The guidelines suggested by the authors in this section are similar in content and spirit to the American Psychiatric Association's recommendations listed at the end of the foreword. Memories of trauma, especially those that were repressed, should be taken seriously but not at face value. Distortion of memory is not uncommon, but error in some areas does not imply error in all. Research is needed to link what is known about memory processing to the effects of trauma on memory. Also, the role of memory retrieval and working through in the psychotherapy of trauma requires further empirical exploration: must one remember in order to forget? These chapters combine the cold light of investigation with the empathic warmth of clinical care. Sullivan defined psychotherapy as "participant observation." The therapist must participate in a real and caring relationship but always be able to step back and observe what is happening in it. Therapists must be neither credulous nor calculating: don't forget.